ADVANCES IN
MEDICAL ONCOLOGY, RESEARCH
AND EDUCATION

Volume III

EPIDEMIOLOGY

ADVANCES IN MEDICAL ONCOLOGY, RESEARCH AND EDUCATION

Proceedings of the 12th International Cancer Congress,
Buenos Aires, 1978

General Editors: A. CANONICO, O. ESTEVEZ, R. CHACON and S. BARG, Buenos Aires

Volumes and Editors:

(Each volume is available separately.)

Pergamon Journals of Related Interest

ADVANCES IN ENZYME REGULATION
COMPUTERIZED TOMOGRAPHY
EUROPEAN JOURNAL OF CANCER
INTERNATIONAL JOURNAL OF RADIATION ONCOLOGY, BIOLOGY, PHYSICS
LEUKEMIA RESEARCH

ADVANCES IN MEDICAL ONCOLOGY, RESEARCH AND EDUCATION

Proceedings of the 12th International Cancer Congress,
Buenos Aires, 1978

Volume III

EPIDEMIOLOGY

Editor:

JILLIAN M. BIRCH

Department of Epidemiology and Social Research
Christie Hospital and Holt Radium Institute
Manchester

PERGAMON PRESS

OXFORD · NEW YORK · TORONTO · SYDNEY · PARIS · FRANKFURT

U.K.	Pergamon Press Ltd., Headington Hill Hall, Oxford OX3 0BW, England
U.S.A.	Pergamon Press Inc., Maxwell House, Fairview Park, Elmsford, New York 10523, U.S.A.
CANADA	Pergamon of Canada, Suite 104, 150 Consumers Road, Willowdale, Ontario M2J 1P9, Canada
AUSTRALIA	Pergamon Press (Aust.) Pty. Ltd., P.O. Box 544, Potts Point, N.S.W. 2011, Australia
FRANCE	Pergamon Press SARL, 24 rue des Ecoles, 75240 Paris, Cedex 05, France
FEDERAL REPUBLIC OF GERMANY	Pergamon Press GmbH, 6242 Kronberg-Taunus, Pferdstrasse 1, Federal Republic of Germany

First edition 1979

British Library Cataloguing in Publication Data

International Cancer Congress,
12th, Buenos Aires, 1978
Advances in medical oncology, research and
education.
Vol.3: Epidemiology
1. Cancer
I. Title II. Canonico, A
III. Birch, Jillian M
616.9'94   RC261   79-40693
ISBN 0-08-024386-X
ISBN 0-08-023777-0 Set of 12 vols.

In order to make this volume available as economically and as rapidly as possible the authors' typescripts have been reproduced in their original forms. This method unfortunately has its typographical limitations but it is hoped that they in no way distract the reader.

*Printed and bound at William Clowes & Sons Limited
Beccles and London*

Contents

Foreword

This book contains papers from the main meetings of the Scientific Programme presented during the 12th International Cancer Congress, which took place in Buenos Aires, Argentina, from 5 to 11 October 1978, and was sponsored by the International Union against Cancer (UICC).

This organisation, with headquarters in Geneva, gathers together from more than a hundred countries 250 medical associations which fight against Cancer and organizes every four years an International Congress which gives maximum coverage to oncological activity throughout the world.

The 11th Congress was held in Florence in 1974, where the General Assembly unanimously decided that Argentina would be the site of the 12th Congress. Argentina was chosen not only because of the beauty of its landscapes and the cordiality of its inhabitants, but also because of the high scientific level of its researchers and practitioners in the field of oncology.

From this Assembly a distinguished International Committee was appointed which undertook the preparation and execution of the Scientific Programme of the Congress.

The Programme was designed to be profitable for those professionals who wished to have a general view of the problem of Cancer, as well as those who were specifically orientated to an oncological subspeciality. It was also conceived as trying to cover the different subjects related to this discipline, emphasizing those with an actual and future gravitation on cancerology.

The scientific activity began every morning with a Special Lecture (5 in all), summarizing some of the subjects of prevailing interest in Oncology, such as Environmental Cancer, Immunology, Sub-clinical Cancer, Modern Cancer Therapy Concepts and Viral Oncogenesis. Within the 26 Symposia, new acquisitions in the technological area were incorporated; such acquisitions had not been exposed in previous Congresses.

15 Multidisciplinary Panels were held studying the more frequent sites in Cancer, with an approach to the problem that included biological and clinical aspects, and concentrating on the following areas: aetiology, epidemiology, pathology, prevention, early detection, education, treatment and results. Proferred Papers were presented as Workshops instead of the classical reading, as in this way they could be discussed fully by the participants. 66 Workshops were held, this being the first time that free communications were presented in this way in a UICC Congress.

The Programme also included 22 "Meet the Experts", 7 Informal Meetings and more than a hundred films.

METHODOLOGY

The methodology used for the development of the Meeting and to make the scientific works profitable, had some original features that we would like to mention.

The methodology used in Lectures, Panels and Symposia was the usual one utilized in previous Congresses and functions satisfactorily. Lectures lasted one hour each. Panels were seven hours long divided into two sessions, one in the morning and one in the afternoon. They had a Chairman and two Vice-chairmen (one for each session). Symposia were three hours long. They had a Chairman, a Vice-chairman and a Secretary.

Of the 8164 registered members, many sent proferred papers of which over 2000 were presented. They were grouped in numbers of 20 or 25, according to the subject, and discussed in Workshops. The International Scientific Committee studied the abstracts of all the papers, and those which were finally approved were sent to the Chairman of the corresponding Workshop who, during the Workshop gave an introduction and commented on the more outstanding works. This was the first time such a method had been used in an UICC Cancer Congress.

"Meet the Experts" were two hours long, and facilitated the approach of young professionals to the most outstanding specialists. The congress was also the ideal place for an exchange of information between the specialists of different countries during the Informal Meetings. Also more than a hundred scientific films were shown.

The size of the task carried out in organising this Congress is reflected in some statistical data: More than 18,000 letters were sent to participants throughout the world; more than 2000 abstracts were published in the Proceedings of the Congress; more than 800 scientists were active participants of the various meetings.

There were 2246 papers presented at the Congress by 4620 authors from 80 countries.

The Programme lasted a total of 450 hours, and was divided into 170 scientific meetings where nearly all the subjects related to Oncology were discussed.

All the material gathered for the publication of these Proceedings has been taken from the original papers submitted by each author. The material has been arranged in 12 volumes, in various homogenous sections, which facilitates the reading of the most interesting individual chapters. Volume XII deals only with the abstracts of proffered papers submitted for Workshops and Special Meetings. The titles of each volume offer a clear view of the extended and multidisciplinary contents of this collection which we are sure will be frequently consulted in the scientific libraries

We are grateful to the individual authors for their valuable collaboration as they have enabled the publication of these Proceedings, and we are sure Pergamon Press was a perfect choice as the Publisher due to its responsibility and efficiency.

Argentina   Dr Abel Canónico
March 1979   Dr Roberto Estevez
                                 Dr Reinaldo Chacon
                                 Dr Solomon Barg

                                 General Editors

Introduction

This volume deals with epidemiology in its broadest sense. A common theme in many of the papers is the emphasis on the very wide scope for research and the need for trained research workers in this expanding branch of oncology. This point is discussed particularly in relation to the countries of Latin America.

An important development in epidemiology is the greater use of laboratory studies in parallel with traditional techniques. Sero-epidemiological investigations relating to potential oncogenic viruses and metabolic studies on environmental carcinogens are included.

The interaction between genetic and environmental factors is discussed and some important data on occupational carcinogenesis is presented.

JILLIAN BIRCH
March 1979

Cancer Epidemiology

Panel Chairman's Summary

Gregory T. O'Connor
Co-Chairman: **Nubia Muñoz**

Symposium No. 14 on Cancer Epidemiology was opened by the Chairman, Dr. G. T. O'Conor, who emphasized the need for research which focuses on hypotheses concerned with etiologic mechanisms. Epidemiologic research must progress beyond the establishment and refinement of demographic associations between cancer types and environmental factors to those sorts of investigations which utilize a multidisciplinary approach including application of the newest laboratory technology.

The Symposium was divided into four parts. The first two sections dealt with specific aspects of tumor biology in which epidemiologic techniques can be effectively applied: 1) precancerous lesions and 2) diet and nutrition. In the third section a presentation and discussion of an ongoing study on colon cancer proved to be a superb illustration of how a well managed multidisciplinary approach can yield new and relevant information. In the fourth section several epidemiologists from Latin America outlined and discussed the opportunities for etiologic studies which exist in virtually all of the countries of Latin America.

Dr. C. Cuello from Cali, Colombia presented morphological evidence for the relationship of thyroid adenomas to endemic parenchymatous nodular goiter. These adenomas which represent a neoplastic proliferation of thyroid cells are of high incidence in areas where goiter is endemic. They also have a higher prevalence in patients with the follicular and anaplastic types of thyroid cancer than in the general population or in patients with papillary or medullary carcinomas.

Dr. C. Marigo from Sao Paulo, Brazil and Dr. E. Sato from Kagoshima, Japan have extended previous studies which confirm that epithelial dysplasia of the esophagus, stomach, and large bowel are precancerous changes in these organs. In the stomach the epithelial changes occur in sites where intestinal metaplasia has occurred and in the colon in association with formation of adenomatous polyps. The degree of dysplasia at all sites can be estimated on a morphological basis or by measurement of DNA content. The frequency of these changes as seen in surgical, as well as autopsy material (including Coroner's cases) correlates with the incidence of invasive cancer at these sites in both high and low risk populations. The similarity of observations in Brazil and Japan give further emphasis to the fact that the microenvironment in which

3

precancerous lesions develop provides special opportunities for analysis of
the effects of environmental factors which are not possible in population
studies.

In the section on nutrition, Dr. L. Kinlen from Oxford, England described his
studies in nuns and in vegetarians. These population groups have lower
incidence and mortality rates for cancers at certain sites. His comments,
however, and those of the discussants stressed the problems inherent in the
interpretation of these types of studies in respect to choice of controls
and multifactorial influences.

Dr. F. de Waard from Utrecht, The Netherlands briefly reviewed the evidence for
the relation of diet and nutrition to cancer. He pointed out that the etiology
of cancer is more complex than just the introduction of a carcinogen into our
food. Existing knowledge and favored hypotheses suggest an interplay between
extrinsic factors, whether they be naturally occurring or artificially introduced, and a variety of host factors. Professor de Waard has had a special
interest in the effect of overnutrition or obesity on breast and endometrial
cancer. He and his colleagues have shown the relationship between obesity
and extraovarian estrogen production. They are testing hypotheses in the
laboratory and by means of intervention studies which link diet and its effect
on steroid metabolism with cancers of the breast, ovary, endometrium, colon,
and prostate.

Dr. G. Williams from New York, USA, extended the discussion of diet and cancer
into the next section of the Symposium by describing in some detail the multidisciplinary studies being carried out on colon cancer by the group at the
American Health Foundation. They have shown that high risk groups in different
countries, but on a Western-type diet, display increased amounts of fecal bile
acid and cholesterol metabolites, increased concentration of intestinal
anaerobic bacteria and fecal mutagens. In addition one low risk group studied
has increased fecal bulk due to dietary fiber content. Extension of these
observations to laboratory studies has shown that rats on a high fat diet are
more susceptible to colon tumor induction, excrete greater quantities of bile
acids and neutral sterols, and that certain bile acids act as tumor promoters.
All these results support the role of dietary fat as a source of tumor promoters
and suggest an antagonistic role for fiber. Dr. D. Thomas of Seattle, Washington
USA, discussed the foregoing paper and outlined the activities of the Breast
Cancer Task Force of the U.S. National Cancer Institute as another example of
a coordinated multidisciplinary approach to cancer epidemiology. The ultimate
objective of these programs dealing with biologic mechanisms is to develop the
knowledge base which will permit the rational design of preventive measures.

In the final part of the Symposium, Dr. J. deSouza from Sao Paulo, Brazil,
Dr. N. Munoz from Lyon, France, and Dr. P. Correa from New Orleans, Louisiana,
USA, described ongoing, as well as projected studies in Latin America which
are directed to specific problems existing in this part of the world. Gastric
cancer and the role of N-nitroso compounds are being investigated in several
high and low risk areas. Latin American coutries with very high rates of
cervical cancer provide a unique opportunity to evaluate screening effects,
as well as to carry out seroepidemiological and other types of studies which
may be expected to provide new information on the natural history of the
disease.

Ethnic as well as specific environmental factors for a number of other cancer
types can be studied with advantage in Latin American countries which show
widely different and variable incidence patterns.

Dr. deSouza suggested some general guidelines for encouraging epidemiology
research in Latin America.

1. Short courses in cancer epidemiology for pathologists, clinicians, and
   surgeons to be sponsored by the appropriate University Medical School
   Departments.

2. Better selection of candidates for Schools of Public Health--opportunity
   for training should not be limited to "employees of health agencies."

3. Government agencies should support research teams associated with teaching
   institutions.

4. Funding for research projects should include fellowship support in order
   to encourage the development and training of epidemiologists.

5. International collaboration should be expanded.

Epidemiological Opportunities in Latin America

Nubia Muñoz

International Agency for Research on Cancer, Lyon, France

ABSTRACT

Some of the opportunities for epidemiological research in Latin America are discussed. Two approaches are used in the pinpointing of these special situations:
1. The identification of populations with high or low rates for specific types of cancer. Using data from "Cancer Incidence in Five Continents" and the Inter-American Investigation of Mortality, research opportunities in cancer of the cervix, stomach, lung, penis, and other tumours are reviewed. 2. The identification of population groups exposed to known carcinogens or risk factors. Among the known carcinogens to which humans are exposed, some pesticides are of special interest in view of their widespread use in many Latin American countries. Follow-up studies of population groups occupationally exposed to those pesticides will be of great value in the estimation of their carcinogenic risk for humans.

Key words: Epidemiology: Cervical Cancer: Gastric Cancer: Pesticides.

Cancer is increasingly recognized in Latin America as an outstanding health problem. The Inter-American Investigation of Mortality has shown that cancer is the first or second cause of death at ages 15-74 in ten Latin American cities (Puffer and Griffith, 1967). The growing awareness of the magnitude of the cancer problem is shown by the establishment of a number of cancer divisions or advisory councils in the Ministries of Health in Latin America, by the launching of national campaigns against cancer, and by the establishment of national cancer plans to concentrate resources in the field of cancer treatment and education.

Two approaches could be used in the pinpointing of opportunities for epidemiological research in Latin America. Firstly, the identification of populations with high or low rates for specific types of cancer. Secondly, the identification of population groups exposed to known carcinogens or risk factors. Some of these opportunities will be reviewed.

POPULATIONS WITH HIGH OR EXCEPTIONALLY LOW RATES FOR CERTAIN TYPES OF CANCER

Data from "Cancer Incidence in Five Continents", Vol. III (1976) and from the Inter-

7

American Investigation of Mortality (Puffer and Griffith, 1967) are used to identify the following malignant tumours which have striking variations within Latin
America, as shown in Tables 1 and 2.

Gastric Cancer

High incidence rates are observed in Sao Paulo (Brazil) and Cali (Colombia); intermediate rates for Jamaica, Recife (Brazil) and Puerto Rico, and low rates for Cuba
(Table 1).   In the mortality study high death rates were found in Bogota,
Guatemala City, Riberao Preto and Santiago, and an extremely low rate was reported
in Mexico City (Table 2).   Marked intra country differences have been described in
Colombia and Chile (Muñoz and others, 1968; Medina, 1973).   These contrasting
situations are being used in different epidemiological studies, mainly to evaluate
the role of N-nitroso compounds or their precursors in the development of gastric
cancer (Cuello and others, 1976; Armijo and Coulson, 1975).

Cervical Cancer

Very high incidence rates for cervical cancer are observed in Cali (Colombia),
Recife (Brazil) and Jamaica.   Sao Paulo (Brazil), Puerto Rico and Cuba have intermediate rates (Table 1).   High death rates are reported from Lima (Peru), Mexico
City, Guatemala City, Santiago (Chile), Caracas (Venezuela) and Bogota (Colombia);
intermediate death rates for Sao Paulo and Riberao Preto in Brazil, and La Plata in
Argentina (Table 2).   Although the epidemiological evidence indicates that this
cancer is related to sexual intercourse, and a venereally transmitted agent has been
postulated as the cause, the nature of this agent is still unknown.   Among the
candidate agents three viruses have been postulated: herpes simplex type 2, cyto-
megalovirus and papilloma virus.   The evidence linking these viruses to cervical
cancer remains inconclusive (Muñoz, 1973; Rawls, Adam and Melnick, 1972), and there
are still many technical difficulties associated with such studies which remain to
be resolved.   In the absence of a promising aetiological hypothesis which would
make primary prevention possible in the near future, research efforts in developing
countries should therefore be directed towards early detection.   After a long-
standing controversy on the value of screening programmes for cancer of the cervix,
only recently, in well-conducted screening programmes in Canada, Iceland and Finland
(Timonen, Nieminen and Kauraniemi, 1974; Walton and others, 1976; Johannesson,
Geirsson and Day, 1978), has convincing scientific evidence been produced which
indicates that screening is effective in reducing the mortality for cervical cancer.
Screening campaigns for cervical cancer are under way in most Latin American countries
but with inadequate planning and evaluation.   To maximize the benefit and to
minimize the cost of these screening programmes, an understanding of the natural
history of cervical cancer is essential.   Although numerous estimates of the average
duration of the pre-invasive disease have been made, this is not the crucial factor
to consider in the design of a screening programme.   What it is necessary to assess
is the proportion of invasive cancers which pass through the in situ phase slowly
enough to be easily detected and, as opposed to those, the proportion which pass so
quickly that no realistic programme will detect them.

It is unlikely that the natural history of cervical cancer in the high-risk populations of Latin America is different from the natural history of this disease in
the low-risk populations of Europe and North America.   This is supported by the
different patterns of the age distribution curves in high and low-risk populations
(Muñoz, 1973).   The first step will be, therefore, to determine the distribution
of duration of the pre-invasive phase in a high-risk population in Latin America,
which will then make it possible to formulate a series of practical recommendations
similar to those contained in the Walton Report (1976).

Cancer of the Penis

Relatively high incidence rates for this tumour are reported from Recife (Brazil), Jamaica and Puerto Rico (Table 1). A viral aetiology has been postulated also for this tumour, but few epidemiological studies have been carried out to test this hypothesis. This may be an area which warrants further attention.

Cancer of the Lung

The high incidence rates in Cuba, both for males and females, are outstanding when compared with the rest of Latin American registries (Table 1). The same is true for La Plata, when the death rates are analyzed (Table 2). A case-control study on lung cancer and smoking habits has been sponsored in Cuba. In a survey on smoking patterns in Latin America, La Plata showed the highest proportion of cigarette smokers in males (58%) among the eight cities included in the study. Among the male cigarette smokers in this city, 38% smoke 20 or more cigarettes per day, 65% smoke blond cigarettes and 76% inhale the smoke deeply (Joly, 1977).

Other Cancers

La Plata also shows relatively high death rates for cancer of the bladder, colon, oesophagus and larynx when compared with the rest of Latin American cities (Table 2). Sao Paulo has the highest reported incidence rate for cancer of the larynx and a relatively high incidence rate for cancer of the oesophagus (Table 1). These special situations have motivated several epidemiological studies on precancerous lesions of the oesophagus, larynx and colon, and these are under way in La Plata and Sao Paulo.

IDENTIFICATION OF POPULATION GROUPS EXPOSED TO KNOWN CARCINOGENS OR RISK FACTORS

Relatively few risk factors which are recognized as causally associated with human cancer have been identified. These are smoking, alcohol drinking, certain sexual and reproductive patterns and some dietary habits. However, their exact role and mode of action are not known. On the other hand, a number of chemical agents known to be carcinogenic in experimental animals and to which humans are exposed have been identified. A total of 368 chemicals have been evaluated for their carcinogenic risk in a special programme of the International Agency for Research on Cancer (Tomatis and others, 1978). Of these, 26 have been associated with cancer induction in humans. For 221 chemicals some evidence of carcinogenicity was found in experimental animals, and for the remaining 121 chemicals the available data were inadequate for evaluation. The three main uses of, or exposures to, these chemicals are, industry, drugs and pesticides. Although occupational exposures to some industrial chemicals may be of importance in certain areas of Latin America, the exposure to pesticides is likely to affect a greater proportion of the population. The rate of growth of pesticide use in developing countries has been described in a FAO report (Arnold, 1975). The estimated use in seven South American countries in 1975 was as high as 72,000 metric tons. Toxicity from pesticides has been described in several Latin American countries (Davies, 1978), but the long term effects of exposure to pesticides are unknown. These are of special interest, in view of the fact that several pesticides are known to be carcinogenic for experimental animals (Tomatis and others, 1978). Follow-up studies of population groups with a widespread occupational exposure to pesticides will be of great value in the evaluation of their carcinogenic risk for humans. These studies could be implemented in some Latin American countries.

TABLE 1 Age-standardized Incidence Rates per 100,000 Population
for Selected Cancers in Latin America

Cancer Registries	Gastric Cancer		Genital Cancer		Lung Cancer		Laryngeal Cancer		Oesophageal Cancer	
	Males	Females	Cervix	Penis	Males	Females	Males	Females	Males	Females
CALI	44.5	26.3	62.8	2.0	18.6	5.1	6.5	1.6	2.8	1.3
CUBA	14.3	7.3	19.5	1.4	44.7	16.1	8.5	1.4	5.7	2.4
JAMAICA	25.2	11.1	40.4	6.4	21.2	5.0	3.7	0.4	9.1	4.7
PUERTO RICO	23.3	10.1	25.6	4.6	15.4	5.0	6.4	1.4	14.8	5.4
RECIFE	24.3	10.8	58.1	6.8	15.7	5.6	8.5	0.9	5.2	1.6
SAO PAULO	49.5	21.5	27.5	2.9	25.0	5.1	14.1	1.2	13.1	2.2

Waterhouse, J., Muir, C., Correa, P. and Powell, J.   Cancer Incidence in Five
Continents, Vol. III, 1976

TABLE 2   Age-standardized Death Rates per 100,000 Population
for Selected Cancers in Latin America

CITIES	Gastric Cancer		Cancer of the Cervix	Lung Cancer		Bladder Cancer		Colon Cancer	
	Males	Females		Males	Females	Males	Females	Males	Females
BOGOTA	45.2	38.4	19.3	9.1	3.5	3.4	1.6	1.5	2.7
CALI	33.8	14.7	43.5	8.8	2.9	3.9	2.1	2.7	2.5
CARACAS	27.6	14.2	20.5	24.0	5.7	7.5	0.4	4.2	2.6
GUATEMALA CITY	34.6	24.4	25.5	6.0	2.0	3.4	0.9	1.8	2.5
LA PLATA	20.8	10.9	8.6	59.0	2.9	14.6	0.5	7.8	7.8
LIMA	30.3	21.3	38.2	17.9	5.5	2.3	1.5	3.9	3.4
MEXICO CITY	8.3	5.8	27.8	7.8	2.2	3.6	0.4	2.6	2.0
RIBERAO PRETO	41.8	16.0	11.1	9.4	6.1	6.5	-	4.1	3.8
SANTIAGO	38.3	19.5	21.0	23.7	5.0	1.3	0.3	2.2	2.4
SAO PAULO	26.0	17.0	12.4	14.8	2.9	3.6	0.7	4.1	4.9

Puffer, R.R. and Griffith, G.W. (1967).   Patterns of Urban Mortality - Report of the Inter-American Investigation of Mortality.   Pan American Health Organization Scientific Publication No. 151.

Armijo, R. and Coulson A.H. (1975). Epidemiology of stomach cancer in Chile - The role of nitrogen fertilizers. Int. J. Epid., 4, 301-309.

Arnold, F. T. (1975). International demand and supply for chemical pesticides with analysis and predictions for developing coutries. FAO Survey .

Cuello, C., Correa, P., Haenszel, W., Gordillo, G., Brown, C., Archer, M. and Tannenbaum, S. (1976). Gastric cancer in Colombia. I. Cancer risk and suspect environmental agents. J. natl Cancer Inst. 57, 1015-1020.

Davies, J. (1978). Personal communication.

Johannesson, G., Geirsson, G. and Day, N. (1978). The effect of mass screening in Iceland, 1965-74, on the incidence and mortality of cervical carcinoma. Int. J. Cancer, 21, 418-425.

Joly, D. J. (1977). El habito de fumar en America Latina - Informe de una encuesta realizada en ocho ciudades en 1971. Organizacion Panamericana de la Salud. Publicacion Cientifica No. 337.

Medina, E. (1973). Variaciones geograficas y cronologicas del cancer gastrico en Chile. Rev. Med. Chile, 101, 574-581.

Muñoz, N., Correa, P., Cuello, C. and Duque, E. (1968). Histologic types of gastric carcinoma in high and low-risk areas. Int. J. Cancer, 3, 809-818.

Muñoz, N. (1973). Virological and endocrinological aspects of carcinoma of the uterine cervix. In: W. Nakara, T. Hirayama, K. Nishioka and H. Sugano (Eds.), Analytic and experimental epidemiology of cancer, University of Tokyo Press, Tokyo. pp. 51-61.

Muñoz, N., de-Thé, G., Aristizabal, N., Yee, C., Rabson, A. and Pearson, G. (1975). Antibodies to herpesviruses in patients with cervical cancer and controls. In: G. de-Thé, M.A. Epstein and H. zur Hausen (Eds.), Oncogenesis and Herpesviruses II, International Agency for Research on Cancer, Lyon. (IARC Scientific Publications No. 11). pp. 45-51.

Puffer, R. P. and Griffith, G. W. (1967). Patterns of urban mortality. Pan American Hlth Org. Scientific Pub. No. 151.

Rawls, W. E., Adam, E. and Melnick, J. L. (1972). Geographical variation in the association of antibodies to herpesvirus type 2 and carcinoma of the cervix. In: P.M. Biggs, G. de-Thé and L.N. Payne (Eds.), Oncogenesis and Herpesviruses I, International Agency for Research on Cancer, Lyon. (IARC Scientific Publications No. 2). pp.424-427.

Timonen, S., Nieminen, U. and Kauraniemi, T. (1974). Mass screening for cervical carcinoma in Finland. Organization and effect on morbidity and mortality. Ann. chir. gynaec. Fenn. 63, 194-112.

Tomatis, L., Agthe, C., Bartsch, H., Huff, J. Montesano, R., Saracci, R., Walker, E. and Wilbourn, J. (1978). Evaluation of the carcinogenicity of chemicals: A review of the monograph program of the International Agency for Research on Cancer. Cancer Res. 38, 877-885.

Walton, R. J., Blanchet, M., Boyes, D. A., Carmichael, J. A., Marshall, K. G., Miller, A. D., Thompson, D. W., and Hill, G. B. (1976). The Walton Report: Cervical cancer screening programs. Can. med. Ass. J. 114.

Waterhouse, J., Muir, C., Correa, P., Powell, J. and Davis, W. (Eds.),(1976). Cancer Incidence in Five Continents, Vol. III. International Agency for Research on Cancer, Lyon. (IARC Scientific Publications, No. 15).

Opportunities for Research on Cancer Epidemiology in Latin America

Pelayo Correa

Professor of Pathology, Louisiana State University Medical Center,
1542 Tulane Avenue, New Orleans, Louisiana, U.S.A.

ABSTRACT

Cancer epidemiology studies in Latin America are put in perspective by analyzing the health and demographic conditions. Examples of opportunities for epidemiologic studies are given. The main obstacles to research are pointed out and several approaches to epidemiologic studies discussed.

KEYWORDS: epidemiology, research, Latin America

INTRODUCTION

Latin America is a rather vague, general term applied to American countries with a strong cultural background of Mediterranean-European origin. Some Central and South American communities, such as Jamaica and the Guianas, are predominantly of English, Dutch, or other cultural backgrounds while others, such as the Spanish-speaking populations of Texas and New Mexico, which would qualify for the term, are not included in the group for reasons of political-administrative-geographic boundaries. Our remarks are directed mainly to those countries with a strong racial and cultural Spanish or Portuguese (Iberic) roots, mainly reflected in the official language of the country.

It should be understood that there is a great racial and socioeconomic diversity in Latin America. Some communities are of almost pure Spanish stock while others are of almost pure Indian stock, frequently within the same country. Similarly, the same country may harbor subpopulations close to the extremes of wealth and poverty. Most of the available national scientific data on health indicators, therefore, represent averages of the contributions of very diverse subpopulations and very few attempts have been made to provide specific data for well-defined, homogeneous subgroups of the population.

A general idea of the health, demographic and economic conditions of the area can be obtained from the data for regional groupings compiled by Logan (1976) as shown in Table 1. Latin America in general is characterized by low gross national product, high birth rates and population growth, high infant mortality, very young populations with high indices of dependency, and inadequate health delivery systems. More recent figures show some improvement in the economic parameters, more tendency to urbanization and a slight decrease in the rate of population growth. The

13

TABLE 1   Health Indicators in the Americas*

	Northern America	Mid-America	Caribbean	Tropical South America	Temperate South America
Area (million km²)	21.5	2.5	0.2	13.7	4.1
Population (millions)	237	79	27	180	39
Population density (per km²)	11	32	114	13	10
Population growth (% per year)	0.9	3.2	1.9	2.9	1.4
Population under 20 years (%)	35	57	51	54	40
Median age of population (years)	29	17	19	18	26
Percent urban population	77	57	48	59	81
Diet: K calories per person per day	3300	2500	2300	2500	2900
Gross national product ($ per capita)	5480	670	680	530	1120
Crude birth rate (per 1000 population)	18	44	35	38	26
Death rate (per 1000 population)	9	10	11	10	9
Expectancy of life at birth (M-F)	69-72	50-65	54-66	53-64	61-69
Infant mortality (per 1000 live births)	18	66	69	90	62
Physicians per 10000 population	15.5	5.1	5.4	5.3	15.2
Nurses and midwives per 10000 population	62.5	7.0	13.9	4.9	5.0
Hospital beds per 10000 population	72.5	12.2	32.6	27.5	48.5

* Source: Logan (1976)

indicators of suboptimal health are more accentuated in the tropical and subtropical areas than in the temperate "southern cone" of the hemisphere. Marked differences in the indices are to be found between specific countries. For example, the Physical Quality Life Index recently developed by the Overseas Development Council and based on life expectancy, literacy and infant mortality shows the following figures for the American Hemisphere: Canada 95, U.S.A. 100, Mexico 73, Guatemala 51, Honduras 51, El Salvador 64, Nicaragua 53, Costa Rica 85, Panama 80, Haiti 32, Dominican Republic 64, Colombia 68, Venezuela 79, Ecuador 67, Peru 59, Brazil 67, Bolivia 43, Paraguay 73, Uruguay 87, Chile 77, Argentina 85.

Epidemiology Resources

The development of cancer research activities in Latin America has been somewhat slow in the past but is picking up speed and broadening in scope in recent years. The earliest studies were based on rather incomplete mortality statistics and on series of cases observed at large hospitals. The mortality data were considerably improved by the special study of the Pan American Health Organization (Puffer and Griffith, 1967). Attempts to organize cancer registries were made some years ago in several countries with some registries in Brazil, Colombia, Cuba and Puerto Rico having been successful over the years. Other registries had a successful initial period and deteriorated afterwards. The registry in Cali, Colombia has led the group. It developed in a collaborative basis of the Universidad del Valle and the Biometry Branch of the National Cancer Institute. Some of the reasons for its success probably have to do with the fact that it has limited its task to an area (the city of Cali) commensurate with its resources, it has had a permanent interest in the utilization of the data and has had adequate consultation facilities with international experts in the field who helped develop the local staff in the early phases of the project. It has developed a collaborative program with Louisiana State University which has led to the extension of the activities of the group to other Latin American countries. The two institutions (LSU and UV) have developed a training program and carried out three workshops on cancer epidemiology especially addressed to Latin American researchers with potential for developing programs in their own countries. The Cali-LSU program is working very closely with the Brazilian and Peruvian registries and has organized new registries in Bolivia and La Plata (Argentina), where especially interesting epidemiological situations have been identified.

Epidemiology research basically depends on the availability of populations with contrasting cancer experience. This is determined by two main forces: genetics and the environment, the latter mainly as it relates to life-style of the individuals. From this standpoint, Latin America offers opportunities that are difficult to match. It would be difficult to find a group of culturally linked countries with more diversity in genetic composition and life-style patterns than Latin America. The other main requisite for epidemiology research is the availability of scientists and trained personnel, mostly epidemiologists, statisticians, and pathologists. Most of the epidemiologists and statisticians in Latin America are not engaged in cancer research. They are mostly concentrating in the field of infectious diseases since it is usually argued that they are more important health problems in the area. Table 1 shows the greatest differential in death rates between developed and developing countries to be in infant mortality. In most cases the etiologic agent related to the immediate cause of death is infectious in nature but other important factors, not fully evaluated to the present time, are the insufficient protection of children by the adult members of the society, a direct result of the high dependency rate of the population. It could then be argued with statistical backing that the prevention of one adult death has more beneficial impact in the community than the prevention of the death of one infant. Cancer is the second most frequent cause of death in adults in most Latin American

countries and its importance as a serious public health problem is gradually being
recognized by the medical and public health profession. Hopefully, this may bring
more researchers and resources into the field of cancer epidemiology.

Cancer Frequency

Table 2 shows examples of age-adjusted incidence rates for populations of Spanish
or Portuguese background appearing in the third volume of Cancer Incidence in Five
Continents. Data for Connecticut, U.S.A. and Miyagi, Japan are included for comparative purposes. Even with the limitations stemming from the limited geographic
areas covered, the available data give a general idea of the distribution of cancer in Latin America and point to the many opportunities for cancer research. The
registries now in operation have limitations, especially in the number of investigators available for analytical studies. In some instances, epidemiologists and
statisticians from schools of public health and departments of preventive medicine
of medical schools are becoming interested in the data and the material of cancer
registries but much more activity in this area is highly desirable.

Some prominent cancer epidemiology peculiarities have been discussed by previous
speakers. Latin America's largest single problem in neoplastic diseases is uterine cervical cancer. This is expected to decline with the preventive measures
being implemented. In females, breast cancer ranks second in frequency. In men,
stomach cancer has been the most frequent in most countries, as exemplified in
Table 3 published by Olper (1975) for Mexico. It shows that lung cancer is gradually becoming the leading cause of death amongst men in large cities. All indicato
are that Mexico (and maybe other Latin American coutries) is on the verge of an
epidemic of lung cancer which has not yet caught the eye of Public Health authorities.

In spite of climatic conditions prevailing in tropical South America, similar to
those of tropical Africa, Burkitt's tumor and hepatocellular carcinomas are relatively rare. An illustration of the variety of cancer patterns is found in
Argentinian data, where cancer distribution resembles more that of Western
European and North American patterns than the Latin American pattern. This is
known mainly through mortality statistics, such as the PAHO study. Particularly
remarkable is the high rate of colon and lung cancer. The incidence of esophageal
and bladder carcinoma are also higher than expected.

Research Approaches

Historically, there have been 3 main kinds of efforts to develop cancer epidemiology studies in Latin America. The first is represented by isolated efforts of
individuals or institutions to develop self-centered programs. There have been
many and very fruitful studies developed on this basis, but their productivity
reaches a peak and then declines or disappears. The second type is "one shot"
international studies based on short-time collection of data and material to be
analyzed in the U.S. or Europe. They provide important and useful data but unfortunately leave very little for the local investigation to build from. The third
type is longitudinal programs based on a long-lasting alliance of Latin American
investigators with investigators based in more developed countries. This allows
the identification of local problems of special interest and the planning and
carrying out of investigations designed to test specific epidemiologic hypotheses.
But most importantly, it allows the development of the local human and material
resources and attracts new talent so as to expect the development of new nuclei
of scientists to carry out independent research. This requires a modest amount of
economic support and provides remedies to the most important obstacle in Latin

TABLE 2 Age-Adjusted (World Population) Incidence Rates of Malignant Neoplasms*

	All Sites Except Skin		Stomach	Colon	Larynx	Lung	Breast	Cervix	Prostate
	Males	Females	Males	Males	Males	Males	Females	Females	Males
Brazil, Recife	181.0	205.1	24.3	2.8	8.5	15.7	41.9	58.1	22.6
Brazil, Sao Paulo	230.6	199.0	49.5	8.7	14.1	25.0	47.3	27.5	16.3
Colombia, Cali	167.7	211.0	44.5	3.2	6.5	18.6	27.8	62.8	19.8
Cuba	169.9	147.0	14.3	6.9	8.5	44.7	28.0	19.5	18.0
Connecticut, USA	285.9	238.1	13.5	30.1	7.8	53.7	71.4	9.8	37.7
New Mexico, USA, Spanish	157.9	177.1	18.6	8.7	2.7	16.7	32.4	21.5	34.3
El Paso, USA, Spanish	192.6	265.0	21.2	9.3	1.6	22.7	52.3	80.9	43.5
Puerto Rico	174.0	146.7	23.3	6.0	6.4	15.4	25.4	25.6	21.4
Japan, Miyagi	184.7	127.7	84.6	5.6	2.0	20.0	13.0	13.8	2.7
Spain, Zaragoza	186.0	133.2	33.8	6.5	12.4	23.5	30.6	4.1	17.7

* Source: Cancer Incidence in Five Continents, Vol. 3, 1976. Selected Populations and Sites.

P. Correa

American research: the isolation of local investigators. We hope that this latter approach will be more often utilized in future research projects in Latin America.

TABLE 3   Frequency Rank of Death Rates for the 5 Most Frequent

Malignant Neoplasms - Mexico*

Rank	1963	1965	1967	1969	1971	1973
			Males - Country			
I	ST	ST	ST	ST	ST	ST
II	PR	PR	PR	LG	LG	LG
III	LK	LK	LK	PR	PR	PR
IV	LF	LF	LG	LK	LK	LK
V	LX	LX	LF	LF	LX	LF
			Males - Federal District			
I	ST	ST	ST	ST	ST	LG
II	PR	LK	LG	LG	LG	ST
III	LK	PR	LK	LK	LK	PR
IV	LF	LF	PR	PR	PR	LK
V	LG	LG	LF	LF	LF	LF

* ST = stomach; LG = lung; PR = prostate; LK = leukemia; LF = lymphoma; LX = larynx

REFERENCES

Logan, W. P. D. (1976). World-health related indicators. World Health Statistics Report, 29, 682-697.
Olper, R. (1975). Epidemiología de las neoplasias. Salud Pública de México, 5, 543-553.
Puffer, R., and G. W. Griffith (1967). Patterns of urban mortality. Pan American Health Organization Publication, No. 151, Washington.

Epidemiological Opportunities in Latin America: Brazil

José Maria Pacheco de Souza

*Departamento Epidemiologia, Faculdade Saúde Pública, Av. Dr. Arnaldo, 715,
Sao Paulo, Brazil*

ABSTRACT

As Latin America in general, Brazil has opportunities for cancer research. At least
two large cities (São Paulo and Porto Alegre) present reliable data on mortality ,
two have registries of cancer in full activity (São Paulo and Recife) and one has
data from a first survey of a registry not thoroughly activated (Rio de Janeiro).
Differences in mortality between São Paulo and Porto Alegre for stomach, lung and
female breast cancers deserve attention for further investigations. As far as
incidence in São Paulo and Recife, some sites present very high incidence when
compared with other places in the world: lip in females, larynx in males, penis,
cervix uteri and stomach are examples. Contrasts in incidence among the Brazilian
cities are pointed out for oesophagus, colon and rectum in male and corpus uteri,
colon and liver in female. Some guidelines are given which may enhance the
broadening of cancer epidemiological research in Brazil.

keywords: cancer epidemiology - Brazil; cancer incidence - Brazil ;
cancer mortality - Brazil.

INTRODUCTION

The infective and parasitic diseases are still highly prevalent in several countries
of Latin America as a consequence of many factors (Table 1).The sanitary authorities
tend, then, to concentrate their efforts in programmes to prevent and/or control
such diseases. The degenerative diseases are not placed as priority. In their study
which included ten cities of Latin America, plus Bristol and San Francisco,
Puffer and Griffith (1967) showed that cancer was clearly also a leading cause of
death in adults (Table 2). Even so, it will take probably some time in the future
for the malignant neoplasms to become a priority in public health. Epidemiology, as
a science in itself, regardless of cancer being or not a priority in public health,
has to play a major role in the search for the discovery of the etiologies and/or
of the risk factors of the malignant neoplasms, in the confirmation of   their
associate "causes", in the proposals for preventive measures and in the evaluation
of the actions for their control. As Latin America in general, Brazil   offers
opportunities for cancer research, although limited in part by the lack of data ,
mainly vital statistics. The cities of Porto Alegre (South of Brazil - 1,000,000
inhabitants) and São Paulo (South East - 7,000,000 inhabitants) present reliable
data on mortality, and the cities of São Paulo, Rio de Janeiro (South East -
6,000,000 inhabitants) and Recife (North East - 1,000,000 inhabitants) have
registries of cancer which allow information in incidence.

MORTALITY

Table 3 uses the available data to compare the cancer death rates for specified sites,

J. M. Pacheco de Souza

in Porto Alegre and São Paulo (it should be mentioned that there are no data according to sexes for Porto Alegre). Using the ratio between the rates of the two cities for each site (the largest as the numerator), it is seen that stomach, lung and female breast deserve attention for further investigation. As far as both Por to Alegre and São Paulo are alike in medical resources and population age structure, differences in mortality data probably reflect diferences in incidence.

Table 1   Annual death rates by infective and parasitic diseases (per 100,000 population) and infant mortality (per 1,000 live born), in some Latin Ame 'rican countries. Around 1974.

COUNTRY	Infanty Mortality	Infective Diseases
Chile	77.1	70.0
Costa Rica	37.6	54.5
Cuba	28.9	21.6
Dominican Rep.	43.4	81.6
Ecuador	70.2	224.6
Honduras	38.9	147.7
Mexico	52.0	137.1
Panama	32.9	78.1
Uruguay	48.6	34.8
Venezuela	46.0	72.6

Source: World Health Statistics Annual: 1977.

Table 2   Annual age-adjusted* death rates from Malignant Neoplasms (per 100,000 population), with percen tages of all deaths, ages 15-74 years, by sex, in each city of the investigation. 1962-1964.

CITY	Death rates		Percentage all death	
	Male	female	Male	Female
Bogotá	115.2	128.0	15.6	20.0
Bristol	155.8	97.3	24.9	28.2
Cali	96.6	120.0	14.5	22.8
Caracas	128.2	114.2	18.1	28.5
Guatemala City	98.0	110.0	13.5	22.0
La Plata	182.6	103.1	27.5	31.0
Lima	112.5	135.5	16.9	28.7
Mexico City	62.2	94.9	8.4	18.9
Ribeirão Preto	137.6	87.1	17.6	17.8
San Francisco	128.2	98.9	19.9	25.8
Santiago	127.6	121.2	13.0	22.8
São Paulo	102.6	95.9	16.2	22.5

* Standard population: the combination of the twelve cities.

Source: PUFFER, R.R. & GRIFFITH,G.W., 1967.

Table 3   Annual cancer death rates for especified sites
(per 100,000 population) in Porto Alegre and São
Paulo and respective ratio (highest rate as the
numerator). Brazil, 1974-76 and 1971-73.

SITE	Death rates Porto Alegre	São Paulo	Ratio
Mouth and pharynx	2.0	2.6	1.3
Oesophagus	5.1	3.7	1.4
Stomach	8.3	17.0	2.0
Large intestine	4.9	5.7	1.2
Rectum	2.1	2.7	1.3
Larynx	2.3	2.5	1.1
Lungs	13.0	8.6	1.5
Breast	17.2	11.6	1.5
Cervix uteri	4.8	3.6	1.3
Uterus	4.6	5.4	1.2
Prostate	7.0	5.2	1.3
All malignant neoplasms	88.2	80.4	1.1

Sources: Secretaria da Saúde do Rio Grande do Sul, 1977a.
Secretaria da Saúde do Rio Grande do Sul, 1977b.
Coordenadoria de Análise de Dados da Secretaria
de Economia e Planejamento do Estado de São Paulo.

Table 4   Annual incidence rates of selected sites in three cities of Bra
zil. Crude and world standardized rates per 100,000 population.
Around 1970.

CITY	São Paulo		Recife		Rio de Janeiro	
SITE (SEX) RATE	Crude	Stand (Rank)	Crude	Stand (Rank)	Crude	Stand
140- Lip (female)	1.2	1.7 (1)	0.9	1.4 (2)	0.4	0.5
141- Tongue (male)	3.7	5.7 (3)	2.6	5.6 (4)	5.4	7.0
143/145- Mouth (male)	4.6	7.0 (3)	3.2	6.9 (4)	6.1	7.8
151- Stomach (male)	29.7	49.5 (4)	11.1	24.3 (31)	9.1	12.4
155- Liver (male)	0.9	1.4 (61)	4.7	10.7 (7)	0.8	1.1
161- Larynx (male)	9.0	14.1 (1)	4.2	8.5 (10)	5.8	7.1
180- Cervix Uteri	22.0	27.5 (15)	38.7	58.1 (3)	27.4	31.0
187.0- Penis	1.8	2.9 (5)	3.5	6.8 (1)	1.7	2.1
174- Breast (female)	36.8	47.3 (43)	26.8	41.9 (48)	20.7	24.0

Sources: SEGI, M., 1977.
Ministério da Saúde - DNC, 1970.
WATERHOUSE, J. and others, 1976.

J. M. Pacheco de Souza

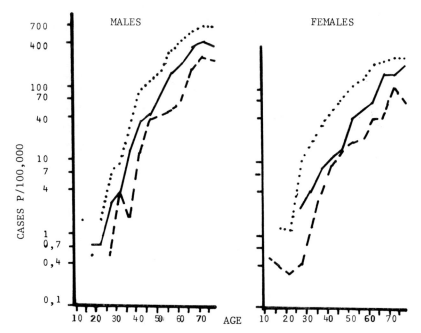

Fig.1.   Age specific incidence of stomach cancer in São Paulo (——),
         Recife (– –) and Okayama (···).
         Source: WATERHOUSE and others, 1976.

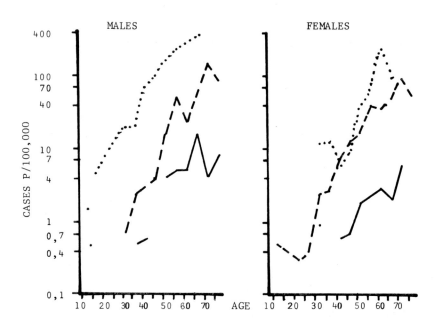

Fig.2.   Age specific incidence of liver cancer in São Paulo (——),
         Recife (– –) and Bulawaio (···).
         Source: WATERHOUSE and others, 1976.

Table 5   Ten most common malignant neoplasms in São Paulo and Recife,their
            annual incidence rates (per 100,000 population) and percentage
            among all malignant neoplasms. Males.

CITY RANK	SÃO PAULO (1969)			RECIFE (1968-1971)		
	SITE	Annual Rate	%	SITE	Annual Rate	%
1	151- Stomach	29.7 (49.5)*	17.5	173- Other Skin	21.6 (41.6)	19.3
2	173- Other Skin	25.5 (41.4)	15.0	151- Stomach	11.1 (24.3)	9.9
3	162- Lung	14.7 (25.0)	8.7	185- Prostate	8.7 (22.6)	7.8
4	161- Larynx	9.0 (14.1)	5.3	162- Lung	7.1 (15.7)	6.3
5	185- Prostate	8.1 (16.3)	4.8	188- Bladder	5.5 (12.4)	4.9
6	150- Oesophagus	7.9 (13.1)	4.7	155- Liver	4.7 (10.7)	4.2
7	188- Bladder	6.8 (12.3)	4.0	161- Larynx	4.2 (8.5)	3.8
8	153- Colon	5.1 (8.7)	3.0	187.0- Penis	3.5 (6.8)	3.1
9	143/145- Mouth	4.6 (7.0)	2.7	143/145- Mouth	3.2 (6.9)	2.9
10	154- Rectum	4.4 (6.9)	2.6	191/192- Brain	2.9 (3.4)	2.6
	All malignant neoplasms	169.3	100	All malignant neoplasms	111.9	100

* In parenthesis the world age standardized rate.

Source: WATERHOUSE, J. and others, 1976.

INCIDENCE

Incidence data may give more leads for research. For some sites, São Paulo and Reci
fe have very high incidence rates as compared with other places in the world,
according to Segi (1977) (Table 4). Table 4 adds also data for these sites from a
first survey of the Cancer Registry of Rio de Janeiro (Ministério da Saúde D.N.C.
1970). The main contrast in risk is for stomach; a second one may be for liver; the
table presents figures only for males, but the contrasts are the same for females.
Investigations in migration and nutrition may be fruitful, when it is known that
São Paulo and Rio de Janeiro have a large population of migrants and of descendants
of migrants and that nutritional deficiency is a problem in Recife (Puffer & Serrano, 1975). Cervix uteri and female breast cancers also deserve attention. It should
be noted that the incidences for breast do not rank high in the world, but both
cervix uteri and female breast are sites with very high incidences among all the
malignant neoplasms in the three cities. Besides this, it was already seen that
breast cancer has a very high mortality. Figures 1 and 2 show incidence   rates
according to age and city for stomach and liver, in each sex, and include similar
data for the city with the highest rate in the world, for comparison (Waterhouse
and others, 1976). It is illustrative to present the ten most common cancers as
they are recorded by the two main registries of Brazil (Waterhouse and others,1976).
Skin is ranked very high for both sexes in São Paulo and Recife. Some sites could
be pointed out for contrasts in incidence, but it seems that oesophagus, colon and
rectum in males and corpus uteri, colon and liver in female deserve closer attention.

Table 6   Ten most common malignant neoplasms in São Paulo and Recife,   their
          annual incidence rates (per 100,000 population) and percentage among
          all malignant neoplasms. Females.

RANK / CITY	SÃO PAULO (1969)			RECIFE (1968-1971)		
	Site	Annual Rate	%	Site	Annual Rate	%
1	174- Breast	36.8 (47.3)*	21.0	180- Cervix uteri	38.7 (58.1)	26.0
2	173- Other Skin	26.2 (37.4)	15.0	174- Breast	26.8 (41.9)	18.0
3	180- Cervix Uteri	22.0 (27.5)	12.6	173- Other Skin	20.8 (36.7)	14.0
4	151- Stomach	14.7 (21.5)	8.4	151- Stomach	5.8 (10.8)	3.9
5	153- Colon	7.3 (10.8)	4.2	155- Liver	5.6 (10.3)	3.8
6	182.0- Corpus Uteri	6.1 (8.5)	3.5	154- Rectum	4.4 (7.7)	3.0
7	154- Rectum	4.9 (7.0)	2.8	183- Ovary	3.5 (5.2)	2.3
8	183- Ovary	4.9 (6.3)	2.8	162- Lung	2.9 (5.2)	1.9
9	162- Lung	3.6 (5.1)	2.1	156- Gallbladder	2.3 (4.1)	1.5
10	156- Gallbladder	1.3 (4.3)	0.7	184- Other Genital	2.2 (3.5)	1.5
	All malignant neoplasms	174.9	100	All malignant neoplasms	149.0	100

* In parenthesis the world age standardized rate.

Source: WATERHOUSE, J. and others, 1976.

EPIDEMIOLOGICAL RESEARCH

In the following, some guidelines are given which may enhance the broadening of
epidemiological research, taking advantage of the opportunities and minimizing the
difficulties in Latin America in general and in Brazil in particular: 1) Departments
of Epidemiology, of Preventive Medicine and of Pathology should provide short
courses in cancer epidemiology to pathologists, clinicians and surgeons.   2)
Alternative criteria for enrollment in Schools of Public Health must be   sought:
future students should not be only "employees of health agencies" or "individuals
with at least X years of experience in public health". 3) The concerned agencies
should concentrate funds in research teams linked to teaching institutions   and
with access to the necessary data. 4) Projects should allocate money for fellow-
ships, in order to recruit future epidemiologists. 5) International cooperation,
colaborative studies and exchange of researchers will prove very useful.

REFERENCES

1.   MINISTÉRIO DA SAÚDE - DNC (1970). O Registro de Câncer da Guanabara, 1968. Di
     visão Nacional do Câncer, Rio de Janeiro 105 pp.
2.   PUFFER, R.R. & GRIFFITH, G.W. (1976). Patterns of Urban Mortality. Pan American
     Health Organization, Washington D.C. (Scientific Publication n.151) 353 pp.
3.   PUFFER, R.R. & SERRANO, C.V. (1975). Patterns of Mortality in Childhood.   Pan

American Health Organization, Washington D.C. (Scientific Publication n.262) 470 pp.

4. SECRETARIA DA SAÚDE DO RIO GRANDE DO SUL (1977). Estatísticas de Saúde: morta-lidade 1970-75.   Porto . vol. 1 - 271 pp.
5. SECRETARIA DA SAÚDE DO RIO GRANDE DO SUL (1977). Estatísticas de Saúde: morta-lidade 1976.   Porto Alegre. vol.2 - 100 pp.
6. SEGI,M. (1977). Graphic Presentation of Cancer Incidence by Site and Area and Population. Segi Institute of Cancer Epidemiology, Nagoya . 42 pp.
7. WATERHOUSE, J., MUIR, C., CORREA,P. & POWELL,J. (Ed.) (1976). Cancer Incidence in Five Continents.   International Agency for Research on Cancer, Lyon. (IARC Scientific Publication n. 15). vol.3 - 584 pp.
8. WORLD HEALTH STATISTICS ANNUAL: 1977 (1977).   World Health Organization, Geneva. vol.1 - 719 pp.

Prevention and Control Program for Cancer of the Cervix in Developing Countries

**João Sampaio Goes Junior and
João Carlos Sampaio Goes**

*Fundação "Centro de Pesquisa de Oncologia", Instituto Brasileiro de Controle
do Cancer, Caixa Postal 11.490, Sao Paulo, Brazil*

Cancer of the cervix is a serious problem in almost every country, but mainly for those in a developing stage.

The diversity which exists in the incidence of the various type of cancer demonstrates the influence that the environmental factors have over it. It is obvious to conclude that it is important to know these factors.

Cervical Cancer is a very serious public health problem for the developing countries: it has one of the highest incidence rates; it attacks women in the most active phase of their lives, when they are still young and necessary to their family and to the community; it has a high correlation with the lower social-economic levels of the population.

When establishing a national program for cancer control, the main problems are the lack of understanding of the true conditions of the developing countries and the lack of medical technology and human resources that they experience.

The lack of understanding of the true conditions is a consequence of the inadequacy of our statistics.There are few registers which are able to give a true and efficient assessment of the problem. Essential data such as incidence, types of cancer, stage of the disease at the moment of diagnosis etc, which are essential for the understanding of the problem, are not quite known. Sixty per cent of the patients who come to the big hospitals of the main cities have the disease in an advanced stage (III or IV). About fifty per cent of these patients come from distant resourceless regions where poverty and low sanitary education are responsible for the high incidence of cervical cancer.

The lack of medical technology and human resources is an even more serious problem in Brazil because of its great expansion (8,511,965 2 km), the number of inhabitants (110,000,000), and the difficulties of transportation. After an accurate evaluation of the situation by means of an assessment made "in loco" of the existing conditions in every specialized body, we established, in all states of the country, an administrative structure with centralized coordination of the National Cancer Division of the Ministry of Health, and decentralized execution. Beginning with 24 Medical Schools, we have now 120 Institutions executing the program.

The Data Bank of the National Cancer Division registered from June 75 to May 77, 60,458 new cases of cancer in both sexes, as shown in the following table:

Region	Male %	Female %
North	33.9	66.1
South	50.7	49.3
North-East	32.6	67.4
South-East	40.6	59.4
Central-West	36.6	63.4
(All Country)	40.2	59.8

The Program provides attendance to private and social welfare patients (N/NCD) and also to the poor patient. The poor patient's attendance is supported by the National Cancer Division of the Ministry of Health (NCD).

Patient's attendance data is shown at the following table:

Region	NCD %	N/NCD %
North	95.9	4.1
South	39.9	60.1
North-East	54.25	45.75
South-East	43.0	57.0
Central-West	14.3	85.7
(All Country)	46.5	53.5

Considering only these cases of highest incidence connected with the female genital system (cancer of the cervix and breast), data collected is as follows:

Region	Cervical Cancer	Breast Cancer
– North	26.4%	9.5%
Amazonas	28.3%	5.9%
Pará	24.6%	13.1%
– North-East	35.4%	11.6%
Ceará	23.2%	16.9%
Piauí	28.0%	9.3%
Rio Grande do Norte	30.8%	12.1%
Maranhão	75.0%	5.3%
Paraíba	26.9%	10.9%
Pernambuco	33.3%	12.6%
Alagoas	33.2%	12.2%
Bahia	33.4%	13.8%
– South-East	16.8%	14.4%
Minas Gerais	14.4%	13.1%
Espírito Santo	19.8%	10.6%
Rio de Janeiro	17.1%	19.7%
São Paulo	15.4%	14.2%
– Central-West	20.4%	9.4%
Goiás	23.8%	11.1%
Mato Grosso	17.0%	7.7%

- South	11.3%	12.4%
Paraná	13.4%	9.4%
Rio Grande do Sul	9.2%	15.5%

Cancer of the Cervix shows highest incidence in the less developed states. On the contrary, the highest incidence of breast cancer is seen in the more developed states.

Migration from the less developed states to the city of São Paulo, which has 10,000,000 inhabitants, is very intensive and continual. The incidence of Cancer of the Cervix is distinctly higher among these newcomers who usually stay in the peripheral area.

The main characteristic of the National Program for Cancer Control is the determination of a modulated structure of the activities so as to permit the collection of standard data from all specialized bodies of the Program. This procedure permits the guidance and direction of all similar activities for development in the various states.

PROCEDURE

The procedure adopted by us since 1972, which we are now proposing as completely feasible, is characterized by the unification of efforts and resources. This policy will avoid duplication of activities in the same area; a duplication which would make the program more expensive for Brazil.

This procedure is as follows:

1. Establishment of an information system to register patient's data such as: name, civil status, race, social welfare situation, age, level of education, and sexual habits.

2. Utilization of the already existing resources, such as Medical Stations, Medical Schools, Institutes, Hospitals, etc.

3. Work centralization in a Central Cytophathology and Pathology Laboratory, and in a Central Hospital.

4. Decentralization of Ambulatory Service in Stations where specimens are collected and first aid is administered, utilizing Federal, State and Municipal Medical Units, located in areas with high population and less economic resources.

5. Utilization of non-medical-technical personnel, specifically trained for first aid and screening.

6. Formation of specialists in all areas of Oncology.

7. Specialized Sanitary Education for the public.

8. Social Welfare Work providing public education, the follow-up of every positive and suspected case, and also treatment.

9. Psychological and physical rehabilitation of the patient who underwent surgery.

We proposed to install a low-cost and profitable standard service to be supplied throughout the entire country for the detection of Cancer of the Cervix.

In 1972, we started a new work procedure working together with the Municipal Government of the city of São Caetano do Sul and the "Instituto Brasileiro de Controle do Cancer (IBCC), assisted by the "Pan American Health Organization (PAHO)" and a special committee of the Secretariat of Health of the State of São Paulo.

In a first screening of 15,000 women, over 20 years of age, 15.14 per thousand suspected and positive cases of Cytology III, IV and V were detected. In a second screening carried out two years later, this result lowered to 3.8 per thousand.

In a 5 years Program, ending in 1977, in a 35,720 women screening, carried out by us in São Caetano, we discovered 757 suspected and positive cases; those cases were properly treated.

A similar program was carried out by us in the city of São Bernardo do Campo, on 23,644 women, and 508 positive and suspected cases were detected.

We can explain the increase in the index of positive cases of cancer observed in São Caetano and São Bernardo as resulting from a better informed public, stimulated by our program in neighboring areas.

Based on the experience obtained, it was possible to establish a useful and feasible work procedure to be carried out in any region of our country or in any other similar developing country.

Together with the cervical cancer research, we performed the breast cancer research according to the same procedure. In a screening of 28,000 women over 20 years of age and without symptoms, 48 cases of carcinoma were detected by us, the incidence rate being 1:550.

Based on this policy and on the experience we had in previous program, we carried out in the peripheral area of São Paulo, an extensive program trying to achieve an attendance of 100,000 women per year; that is, 500 women per day.

From the beginning of its activities till now, the "Instituto Brasileiro de Controle do Cancer (IBCC)" and the "Fundação Centro de Pesquisa de Oncologia (FCPO)" working cooperatively have been carrying out the Peripheral Area Program. We began this Program cautiously and developed it progressively. 83,367 women were submitted to examination being detected 1,207 suspected and positive cases (14,4 per thousand) From this number, 61,798 were examined from May 1977 to April 1978, showing the increase of activities.

Data from the peripheral area program are as follows:

CYTOLOGIC EXAMINATIONS IIIa - 490

		Ic*
Total of suspected or positive biopsies	91	18.6%

Biopsy: Histopathological result	Patients	%
Slight Dysplasia	63	12.9
Moderate Sysplasia	20	4.1
Severe Dysplasia	04	0.8
"In situ" Carcinoma	04	0.8
Invasive Carcinoma	00	0.0
	91	18.6

Negative biopsy (Cervicitis, Metaplasia, Hyperkeratosis, polyp, Reepithelization)	130	26.5
No biopsy made (negative cytology)	269	54.9

*Ic = biopsy / cytology

CYTOLOGIC EXAMINATION   IIIb -   181

		Ic
Total of suspected or positive biopsies	134	74.0

Biopsy:

Histopathological result	Patients	%
Slight Dysplasia	018	9.9
Moderate Dysplasia	083	45.9
Severe Dysplasia	022	12.2
"In situ" Carcinoma	010	5.5
Invasive Carcinoma	001	0.5
	134	74.0

Negative biopsy (Cervivitis, Metaplasia, Hyperkeratosis, Polyp, Reepithelization)

No biopsy made (negative cytology)	016	8.9

CYTOLOGIC EXAMINATION IIIc - 72

		Ic
Total of suspected or positive biopsies	62	86.1

Biopsy:

Histopathological result	Patients	%
Slight Dysplasia	04	5.6
Moderate Dysplasia	13	18.0
Severe Dysplasia	34	47.2
"In situ" Carcinoma	10	13.9
Invasive Carcinoma	01	1.4
	62	86.1
Negative biopsy (Cervicitis, Metaplasia, Hyperkeratosis, Polyp, Reepithelization)	05	7.0
No biopsy made (negative cytology	05	7.0

CYTOLOGIC EXAMINATION   IV -   153

		Ic
Total of suspected or positive biopsies	138	90.2

Biopsy:

Histopathological results	Patients	%
Slight Dysplasia	004	2.6
Moderate Dysplasia	007	4.6
Severe Dysplasia	018	11.8
"In situ" Carcinoma	106	69.3
Invasive Carcinoma	003	1.9
	138	90.2
Negative biopsy (Cervicitis, Metaplasia, Hyperkeratosis, Polyp, Reepithelization)	015	9.8

CYTOLOGIC EXAMINATION   V -   76

		Ic
Total of suspected or positive biopsies	75	87.3

Biopsy:

Histopathological results	Patients	%
Severe Dysplasia	04	4.7
"In situ" Carcinoma	21	24.4
Invasive Carcinoma	44	51.2
Adenocarcinoma of the cervix	06	6.9
	75	87.3
Negative biopsy (Cervicitis, Metaplasia, Hyperkeratosis, Polyp, Reepithelization)	11	12.7

In accordance with the policy of resource coordination which we adopted at the beginning of the program, the "Fundação Centro de Pesquisa de Oncologia (FCPO) and the "Instituto Brasileiro de Controle do Cancer (IBCC)" installed Ambulatories in 23 already-existing Medical bodies of the State and Municipal Governments of São Paulo Patient's preliminary attendance is carried out by the properly trained non-medical personnel, working under the direction and supervision of a responsible doctor.

At this first contact with the patient Level I - both identification data and specimen for cytopathological examination are collected. The cervix is examined and breast palpation is carried out to find tumours, abnormalities or nipple discharge. Following this screening, the suspected cases are sent to the specialized doctor for second level diagnosis.

This screening performed by non medical personnel is very important because it permits mass attendance. In our countries we do not have enough doctors to perform such a task. The accuracy of this kind of screening has already been tested by us, and the results, which were quite satisfactory, have already been published.

We are now extending this screening to the skin and the oral cavity.

Level II attendance is done in the Central Ambulatory by a specialized doctor. Patients are submitted to a complete gynecological examination, Schiler test, colposcopy, and whenever necessary, a biopsy is done.

In Level III of diagnosis, the clinical examination of the breasts is done, including thermography and mammography. Ductography and biopsy are done if necessary.

The training of qualified specialists is essential since there are not enough of them at the moment.

Besides the colposcopy and cytopathology courses for doctors, it is necessary to train qualified cytotechnicians to carry out this program. For that purpose, the "Instituto Brasileiro de Controle do Cancer (FCPO) maintain a regular course for cytotechnicians. This year, the 4th course will certify 15 new cytotechnicians, completing a group of 45.

Other courses such as cytotechnology of the lung, discharge cytology, etc, complement the training for the program.

Public Education informing about the symptoms of cancer must be developed with caution and must be exposed to small groups of people. The information released by television, radio or the press is dangerous. It can cause panic and depression for a quantity of people so large that the possibilities of medical assistance would be exceeded.

According to our program policy, daily lectures are given to people who come to the Central Ambulatory, and also to small community groups, trying to present cancer not as a calamity but as a disease that can be cured when diagnosed early and properly treated.

The Social Assistance Service has a very important task in the program which is to supply information about cancer prevention, to collect data from patients, to take care of the follow up guiding patients to adequate treatment. Letters are sent to patients who, at the screening, showed a suspected or positive case and also visits to their houses are made, inducing them to treatment.

The existence of a Central Ambulatory is essential to guarantee the follow-up of every positive case, reducing to a minimum the loss of contact with patient.

Movable Units providing transitory attendance can be helpful if properly used. We use them as a way of promotion and contact with the surrounding population of small country regions where there is a settled central ambulatory to receive both data and specimen collected from local patients. The movable units should always be limited to small areas under the assistance of the settled ambulatory which is permanently linked with the Central Hospital. We have used this procedure in the small region of the City of Assis, working in a radial distance of 80 km, using a movable unit which is linked to two already installed ambulatories. Two other ones will be installed in a short period of time. So proceeding, it is possible to develop our program in country areas with permanent assistance.

In its first stage, the Assis program performed a 5,422 women attendance, over a 8 month period, detecting 70 suspected cases (12.9 per thousand).

Our experience shows that temporary campaigns utilizing movable medical units throughout the country without the establishment of permanent ambulatories is ineffective and fails in the accomplishment of their tasks. It is absolutely necessary to establish a program which can be permanently carried out in each region, all these regional programs being interlinked and subordinated to the coordination of a central unit which will control all activities.

Nutrition and Cancer, Some Results of Epidemiological Studies

F. de Waard

Institute of Social Medicine, Bijlhouwerstraat 6, University of Utrecht,
The Netherlands

ABSTRACT

Some examples are given of recent progress in our understanding of possible
relationships between nutritional factors and the occurrence of cancer in man.
Particular attention is devoted to cancer of the esophagus, stomach, endometrium
and breast.

There is growing consensus that environmental factors are responsible for 80-90%
of the world-wide variation observed in the cancer incidence in man. However, this
statement is often misunderstood: some non-epidemiologists have been led to believe
that this percentage refers to the proportion of cancers caused by carcinogens
in the air we breathe and the food we eat.
I would like to make it clear that the statement mentioned above uses the word
environment in the broadest sense of its meaning. Thus it includes the various
ways populations live with all their peculiar habits of eating and drinking,
smoking and chewing, in brief: enjoying life.
The ways in which these habits may cause cancer can vary to a large extent.
The most simple mechanism which we can think of, is <u>direct contact of a carcinogen
with the mucosa</u>. In cancer of the digestive tract there is the example of oral
cancer in India where direct contact of the oral mucosa with substances of the
betel nut probably is the dangerous habit.

In the epidemiology of <u>cancer of the oesophagus</u> there has been recent progress.
A large belt of high incidence throughout Central Asia has its Southwestern tail
in Iran near the Caspian sea. A research team of the International Agency for
Research on Cancer (Lyon) has documented large differences in incidence between
neighbouring provinces which are ecologically distinct and where the people have
different life-styles. After years of scientific struggle it now has come to light
that the former nomads of the province of Mazandaran (with the high incidence)
not only smoke opium but also scrape the non-combustible part from their pipes
and swallow it (N.E. Day, pers.comm.).
It is of interest to know that the Bantu-speaking tribes of the Transkei in whom
oesophageal cancer is also quite frequent are fond of pipe-smoking as well.

It will be of interest to learn more about their habit; they seem to cleanse
their pipes taking the "intshongo" into their mouth, but do not swallow it
(Warwick and Harington 1973). Cancer at a particular site can have more than one
cause. In Britanny in the West of France it has been shown by Tuyns and Massé(1973)
in a detailed geographical study that cancer of the oesophagus is highly prevalent
in those regions where strong liquors are preferred rather than wine. These
liquors are often prepared at home, and there is strong suspicion that in this process carcinogens are being introduced in the beverage.

Gastric cancer provides a more complex situation.
It may be that in some places carcinogenic substances are directly introduced
into the stomach. E.g. there is a high incidence in the Northwestern part of
Iceland where seagulls are plentiful; these birds are a delicatessen when singed
over an open fire. (Sigurjonson and Dungal 1967).
However, in the majority of gastric cancer cases the causes may be different.
Epidemiologically speaking there are the following leads: a high incidence in
countries like Japan where salted fish provides a substantial part of the menu;
a low incidence in most tropical countries and a high incidence in Eastern
Europe where winters are long and food preservation a matter of economy;
a declining incidence in affluent countries where food preservation by means of
cooling techniques has been widely introduced. Within some countries a geographic
incidence pattern suggests that soil and fertilisers may be important.
Clinical epidemiologists have noted an increased risk in partially resected
stomachs, in patients with percinious anaemia and other conditions where there
is no acid formation by the gastric mucosa.
These facts could be considered in a new perspective after experimental
oncologists had shown the carcinogenic potential of nitrosamides which can be
formed by the reaction of secondary amines with nitrites.
Secondary amines are abundantly present in fish. Nitrites can be formed out of
nitrates under various conditions but not in the cold nor in the presence of
ascorbic acid (vitamin C). This reaction can be enhanced by bacteria which need a
non-acid environment for their growth. (Correa et al.1975).
Thus there are a number of factors determining the probability of nitrosamide
formation, in the environment as well as in the host. In the 19th century
John Snow knew how to prevent cholera without ever having seen the causal germ.
In the same way we might predict (or speculate at least) that the introduction
of modern food-preserving techniques such as the deep-freeze may be responsible
for the decline in gastric cancer incidence in the United States and parts of
Western Europe (Weisburger and Raineri 1975).

The aetiology of cancer is obviously more complex than just the introduction
of a carcinogen with our food. Further examples of this notion could be given
when treating the epidemiology of colon cancer and of primary cancer of the liver.
However, there is another group of cancers which only recently have been considered
as related to nutrition. The evidence is rather indirect in that these cancers
are much more prevalent among populations suffering from overnutrition, viz. the
inhabitants of North America and Northwestern Europe. This group of cancers
includes those of
                    the mammary glands
                    the endometrium
                    the ovaries
                    the prostate.
Epidemiologists got a bridgehead in their approach by the observations of
clinicians that endometrial cancer is associated with obesity.

The statistical association could be understood after we had detected the relationship between obesity and extra-ovarian estrogen production (de Waard and Oettle 1965, de Waard and Baanders 1969). Mac Donald and Siiteri (1974)and Schindler et al. (1972) provided a firm biochemical basis by showing that the steroid androstenedione can be converted into estrone by peripheral tissues, in particular adipose tissue. Thus the old hypothesis of the dangers of unopposed action of estrogens was revived, and some years later a number of sound epidemiological studies on the association of continuous estrogenic medication with endometrial cancer convinced the experts that the causes of endometrial cancer largely have been unraveled. The following diagram illustrates our present understanding:

	CONTINUOUS SOURCE OF ESTROGENS	+	STATE OF ANOVULATION (NO CYCLE)	
BEFORE MENOPAUSE	OVARIES	+	STEIN-LEVENTHAL OR RELATED SYNDROMES	
				RISK OF ENDOMETRIAL CANCER
AFTER MENOPAUSE	ADIPOSE TISSUE OR ESTROGENIC DRUGS OR CERTAIN OVARIAN TUMORS (RARE)	+	POSTMENOPAUSE	

As we understand things, the reason that the contraceptive pill has not caused endometrial cancer, is because of its rhythm or a built-in progestational phase. Thus the Law of the Sexual Rhythm advanced by Lipschutz as a principle in experimental oncology (Lipschutz 1950) seems to be applicable here.

Needless to say the new knowledge regarding overnutrition and its distant effects has influenced our thinking on the causation of cancer of the breast and the ovary as well. Several studies have been made of a possible relationship between overweight and breast cancer. The issue proved to be somewhat complex because in some studies both weight and height turned out to be risk factors. Positive relationships were found in Brazil, Taiwan, Japan, Poland, Greece, Yugoslavia and Holland. In other countries (United States, Canada, Sweden) no clear association was observed and a Finnish study with negative results lacked the appropriate age-groups of age 60 and over. One methodological reason for the negative findings may be that the range of observed weights in Western countries is fairly restricted. In comparing the Dutch with the Japanese we were struck by the fact thet there is only little overlap between the heaviest Japanese and the lightest Dutch postmenopausal women. If the range of relative risk in the former is about 1.8 and if the same holds for the latter, the gradient of risk with increasing body weight amounts to more than threefold, when considered on a world scale. In other words the proportion of breast cancer incidence observed in five continents that can be attributed to body weight is much larger than anticipated by those who study Western or Eastern populations separately. This is merely an example of the kind of problem we are dealing with in the epidemiology of diseases which are endemic because of overnutrition.

We do not wish to overemphasize the importance of overweight since other parameters of Western nutrition may be important as well. Original concepts as to the cause of ovarian and prostatic cancer may be formulated along lines similar to those concerning cancer of the breast and of the endometrium. As a guideline to our thinking it should be pointed out that cancer of the colon geographically is highly correlated with the three cancers of the female organs mentioned above.

REFERENCES

Correa P., Haenszel W., Cuello C., Tannenbaum S., Archer M., (1975), A model for gastric cancer epidemiology, Lancet 2, 58-59.
Dungal N., Sigurjonsson J., (1967) Gastric cancer and diet, Brit J. Ca 270-276.
Joint Iran-Iarc study group. Oesophageal cancer on the Caspian littoral Lancet 1, 641-642 (1978) and J. Nat.Ca Inst. 59,1127 (1977)
Lipschutz A., Steroid hormones and tumors, Williams & Wilkins Comp., Baltimore (1950)
Mac Donald P.C., Siiteri P.K. (1974) The relationship between the extraglandular production of estrone and the occurrence of endometrial neoplasia Gynec oncol. 2, 259-263.
Schindler A.E., Eberth A., Friedrich E., (1972) Conversion of androstenedione to estrone by human fat tissue. J. clin.endocr.metab. 35, 627-630.
Tuyns A.J., Massé L.M.F. (1973) Mortality from cancer of the oesophagus in Britanny Int.J.Epid. 2, 241-245.
de Waard F., Oettlé A.G. (1965) A cytological survey of postmenopausal estrus in africa. Cancer 18,450-459.
de Waard F., Baanders-van Halewijn E.A., (1969) Cross-sectional data on estrogenic smears in a postmenopausal population. Acta cytol.(Philad,) 13,675-678.
Warwick G.P., Harington J.S. (1973) Some aspects of the epidemiology and etiology of esophgeal cancer with particular emphasis on the Transkei, South Africa Adv.Cancer Res. 17, 81-229, Acad.Press,New York and London.
Weisburger J.H., Raineri R., (1975) Dietary factors and the etiology of gastric cancer.Cancer Res. 35, 3469-3474.

Further Studies on the Etiology of Esophageal Cancer

Department of Chemical Etiology and Carcinogenesis,
Institute of Cancer Research, Chinese Academy of Medical Sciences, Peking,
The People's Republic of China

ABSTRACT

In Linhsien County where esophageal cancer is prevalent, a relatively high level of nitrates, nitrites and secondary amines was found
in the food and the environment. Deficiency of trace element molybdenum in the environment, and the contamination of food by fungi
present a favorable condition for the production of carcinogenic
nitrosamines. A series of experimental studies have been carried out
on the in vivo and in vitro formation of N-nitroso compounds. Secondary amines extracted from local foods have been found to react
readily with $NaNO_2$ to form nitrosamines. Some common fungus species
of Fusarium, Geotrichum, Aspergillus and others not only can reduce
the nitrates to nitrites, but also increased the amount of secondary
amines in contaminated food and promoted the formation of nitrosamines. When small amount of $NaNO_2$ is added to the moldy corn bread,
GC-MS analysis showed the presence of DMNA, DENA, MBNA and a new
compound, N-1-methylacetonyl-N-3-methylbutylnitrosamine. The pickled
vegetables, consumed as a traditional food in Linhsien, have been
heavily contaminated by Geotrichum candidum Link. Animal experiment
indicated the presence of carcinogenic substances in the extract and
concentrated juice of the pickled vegetables and chemical identification is in progress.

DETERMINATION OF NITRATES AND NITRITES IN WATER, SALIVA AND URINE

It is known that nitrates and nitrites are widely distributed in the
environment and that the former can be readily reduced to nitrites
which are the essential components in the synthesis of nitrosamines.
The amount of nitrates and nitrites in water was determined by the
colorimetric method using Griess reagent. Drinking water from 495
wells in the 49 production brigades of Yaotsun Commune were examined
each season in 1976. Nitrates and nitrites were found in most
samples; the concentration was especially high in summer ranging
from 0 to 75 mg/l (average 12.65 mg/l) and 0 to 2.63 mg/l (average
0.052 mg/l) respectively. In fact, the concentration of nitrates in
well water in the 49 brigades during summer showed a positive correlation with the average incidence rate of esophageal cancer for

the years 1969-1972 ($r = 0.233$, $p < 0.05$). Similarly a positive correlation was noted between the incidence rate of marked epithelial
dysplasia, a precancerous lesion of the esophagus, and the nitrate
level in the spring and autumn samples ($r = 0.245$, $p < 0.05$; $r = 0.229$,
$p < 0.05$) and the nitrite content of water taken in autumn ($r = 0.230$,
$p < 0.05$). Further, nitrites in the drinking water used in commune
member's homes - in well water, water stored in jars, warm water in
pots, and liquid food (gruel) - were found in increasing concentration in the order named. For instance, the average concentration of
nitrites in samples taken from warm water pots and gruel were 0.512
mg/l and 0.696 mg/l, respectively, which were 10 to 20 times higher
than those taken from water jars.

Nitrates and nitrites were recovered in the gastric juice and saliva
from Linhsien peasants, but the amount of nitrites in saliva showed
no difference before and after breakfast. A comparative study of
nitrites in saliva carried out among peasants in Linhsien and Hsinyanghsien, a low risk area of esophageal cancer, showed an average
of 4.57 mg/l (216 samples) as against 5.74 mg/l (51 samples). A
significant difference in content of salivary nitrites was observed,
however, between patients with marked epithelial dysplasia or carcinoma of the esophagus and normal controls.

The level of urinary ascorbic acid among inhabitants of Linhsien was
only 1/8 or 1/9 of that among Hsinyanghsien inhabitants. The amount
of nitrites excreted in the urine was markedly diminished following
the administration of vitamin ^{C}, indicating that a low intake of
vitamin ^{C} in Linhsien might have provided a favorable condition for
the formation of nitrosamines from nitrites.

REDUCTION IN NITRATE AND NITRITE CONTENT IN CROPS BY THE USE OF MOLYBDENUM

It is known that the trace element molybdenum is an important constituent of certain enzymes, such as nitrate reductase, and deficiency of molybdenum may lead to the accumulation of nitrates in plants.
Emission spectrometric analysis of food samples from seven counties
in Honan Province showed that the foodstuffs from Linhsien and other
areas with high incidence rate of esophageal cancer contained an
extremely low amount of molybdenum. Catalytic polarography used for
the analysis of molybdenum in the hair, blood serum and overnight
samples of urine showed a much lower amount among the people in Linhsien as compared with those in low risk areas, such as Yuhsien and
Hsinyanghsien counties. There was, besides, a marked difference in
the ratio of copper and molybdenum in the hair taken from Linhsien
and Yuhsien residents, being 161 to 194 and 89 to 101, respectively.
As copper can counteract the physiological action of molybdenum, the
high ratio of these trace elements in Linhsien residents may have
aggravated the effect of molybdenum deficiency. After the application of ammonium molybdate as fertilizer in Linhsien, the molybdenum
content in wheat, maize, millet and rice increased from 0.33-0.48
mg/kg to 0.50-1.49 mg/kg, along with a 25.8-47.8% decrease in nitrate concentration. In vegetables, following the application of
ammonium molybdate, the nitrate and nitrite levels decreased 18.0%
and 27.5% respectively, and the vitamin ^{C} content increased on the
average by 24.8%. Incidentally, the crop yield also increased as a
result of using molybdenum fertilizer.

IN VIVO FORMATION OF N-NITROSO COMPOUNDS FROM PRECURSORS

Since the precursors of nitrosamines are present everywhere, the nitrosation of amines should be considered as the main source in the formation of N-nitroso compounds. In a 170-day experiment, administration of methylbenzylamine and $NaNO_2$ induced esophageal tumors in rats. Further experiment with gavage of sarcosine ester and $NaNO_2$ resulted also in the formation of esophageal carcinoma in all the 21 rats treated for 150-260 days.

In vitro experiment was then carried out on the synthesis of nitrosamines under the influence of the acidity of the gastric juice. It was found that different secondary amines e.g. dimethylamine, diethylamine, methylbenzylamine, could react with $NaNO_2$ to form corresponding N-nitroso compounds in test tubes, containing 5 ml of human gastric juice, at low pH. Furthermore, by feeding pigs with food containing methylbenzylamine or methylphenylamine and $NaNO_2$, we obtained nitrosamine when their stomach contents were analysed at the end of 1-2 hours, though the synthesis of diethylnitrosamine was more difficult owing to the strong basicity of diethylamine. When the secondary amines extracted from the bran of millet or flour of sweet potato, both from Linhsien, were allowed to react with $NaNO_2$ either in test tubes or the rat stomach, nitrosamines formed rapidly. Thus the present experimental results show that the stomach is the principal site for the in vivo formation of N-nitroso compounds from secondary amines and nitrites.

ENHANCEMENT BY FUNGUS IN FORMATION OF NITROSAMINES IN FOOD

In areas where esophageal cancer is prevalent, certain food-stuffs are frequently contaminated by fungus. Our experimental investigation demonstrated that some common species of fungus belonging to Fusarium, Geotrichum, Aspergillus and other genera not only reduced nitrates to nitrites, as has been observed with certain bacteria, but also increased the amount of secondaty amines in food and promoted the formation of nitrosamines. The content of secondary amines in corn bread increased several times after inoculation with Fusarium moniliforme Sheld followed by a few days of incubation. When a small amount of $NaNO_2$ was added to moldy corn bread, GC-MS analysis showed the presence of four N-nitroso compounds, i.e. dimethylnitrosamine (DMNA), diethylnitrosamine (DENA), methylbenzylnitrosamine (MBNA), and a new volatile nitrosamine, N-1-methylacetonyl-N-3-methylbutyl-nitrosamine (MAMBNA), with a molecular weight of 186.13894 (Table 1, Fig. 1). This new compound was synthesized and confirmed by GC-MS, and its amount in contaminated corn bread was estimated as 0.2-0.3 ppm.

Pickled vegetables commonly consumed in Linhsien County which have been found to be heavily contaminated by fungus Geotrichum candidum Link contained high amounts of nitrates, nitrites and secondary amines. The presence of nitrosamines in pickled vegetables is indicated by analysis of thin-layer chromatography, further chemical identification is being carried out. In a preliminary experiment, among 29 rats fed with extracted and concentrated liquid from pickled vegetables for 330 to 730 days, one had adenocarcinoma of the glandular stomach, 4 had fibrosarcoma of the liver and another had angioendothelioma of the thoracic wall, in addition to epithelial

dysplasia in the esophagus and the forestomach. No tumor was noted
in the 10 control rats.

DISCUSSION

In Linhsien County, where the incidence of esophageal cancer is high,
a relatively high level of nitrates, nitrites and secondary amines
has been found in the food and the environment. These precursors
can be readily synthesized to form carcinogenic nitrosamines, especially under the acid condition of the stomach, which may be the
principal site for the formation of this type of carcinogens. De-
fiency of trace element, molybdenum, in the natural environment and
fungus contamination of food may also present favorable conditions
for the production of these carcinogenic substances. The experimental results reported in the present paper show that some fungi
can not only reduce nitrates to nitrites but also decompose proteins
contained in foodstuffs, thus increasing the amount of secondary
amines and promoting the formation of nitrosamines. DMNA, DENA,
MBNA and a new compound, MAMBNA, have been found in corn bread contaminated with Fusarium moniliforme Sheld and some other fungi.
These findings give further information concerning the etiological
factors of esophageal cancer in Linsien County.

Maize is known to contain a rich amount of leucine and isoleucine
which may contribute the basic material, 3-methylbutyl constituent,
for the formation of the new nitrosamine, following the decomposi-
tion of proteins by fungus contamination, while the acetonyl radical
is present in most organisms. Cook (1971) reported that in Africa
a high incidence of esophageal cancer is found in regions where
maize is a staple food, and the consumption of alcoholic drinks made
from maize is considered to be a possible etiological factor. More
recently, Walker et al. (1976) reported the presence of DMNA in
three out of 18 samples of maize beer from southern Africa. Our
present work shows that fungus contamination of maize leads to the
formation of nitrosamines, and among them MBNA is a specific carcinogen which induces esophageal carcinoma in rats.

Much attention is now being paid to the carcinogenic action of certain mycotoxins. Our results demonstrate that in addition to mycotoxins there are chemical carcinogens formed in various moldy foods,
thus opening a new field of research in cancer etiology.

REFERENCES

Cook, P. (1971). Cancer of the oesophagus in Africa. Brit. J.
    Cancer, 25, 853-880.
Editorials (1974). Leads in oesophageal cancer. Lancet, 2, 504.
Sander, J., F. Schweinsberg, and H. P. Menz (1968). Untersuchungen
    über die Entstehung kanzerogener Nitrosamine in Magen. Hoppe-
    Seyler's Z. Physiol. Chem., 349, 1691-1697.
The Coordinating Group for Research on Etiology of Esophageal
    Cancer in North China (1975). The epidemiology and etiology
    of esophageal cancer in North China: A preliminary report.
    Chinese M. J., 3, 167-183.
Walker, E. A., M. Castegnaro, and G. Toussaint (1976). Carcinogens
    in alcoholic beverages. IARC Annual Report, 1976, 53.

TABLE 1 Formation of Nitrosamines in Corn Bread Inoculated with Fungus*

Species of fungus	TLC				GC - M S			
	No. exp.	Positive reaction	Negative reaction	No. exp.	DMNA	DENA	MBNA	MAMBNA
Fusarium moniliforme Sheld	39	34	5	27	1	0	2	24
Aspergillus flavus Link	9	6	3	3	1	2	0	0
A. terreus Thom	4	4	0	2	0	0	0	2
A. niger v. Tiegh	2	2	0	2	1	1	0	0
Geotrichum candidum Link	1	1	0	1	0	0	0	1
Mixed fungi**	4	4	0	4	2	2	0	0
Control	10	1	9	1	1	0	0	0

* Each sample added $NaNO_2$ (1 mg/1 g) after 8-day incubation.

** Mixed fungi: F. moniliforme Sheld, A flavus Link, A. niger v. Tiegh, Penicillium cyclopium Westl. and P. oxalicum Currie et Thom.

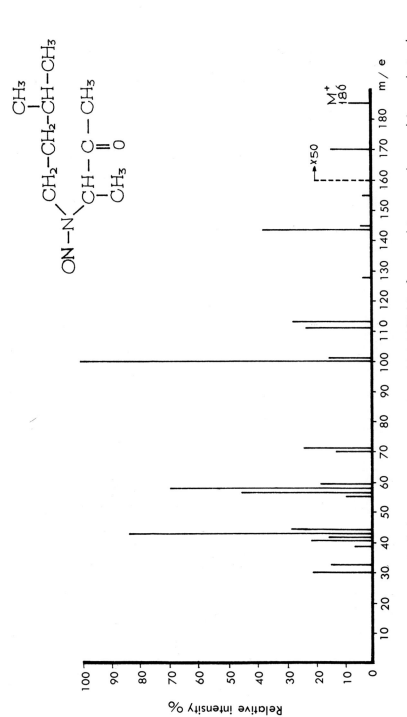

Fig.1   Mass spectrum of the new nitrosamine, MAMBNA, formed in corn bread inoculated with Fusarium moniliforme and added NaNO2.

Factors Associated with Adenocarcinomas of the Large Bowel in Puerto Rico[1]

I. Martínez*, R. Torres**, Z. Frías***, J. R. Colón****, and N. Fernández*****

*Director Cancer Control Program, Department of Health, Puerto Rico
**Director Central Cancer Registry, Cancer Control Program   ***Biometrician
****Assistant Clinical Professor of Medicine, U.P.R., School of Medicine, Puerto Rico
*****Assistant Professor of Biochemistry, U.P.R., School of Medicine, Puerto Rico

[1]Supported by National Cancer Institute Grant 5R26CA14976-2 as part of the National Large Bowel Cancer Project

ABSTRACT

A case-control study of 461 patients with adenocarcinomas of the large bowel was undertaken in Puerto Rico to explore its association with environmental and dietary factors, familial aggregation of cancer, and some personal habits. Four hundred and sixty-one age- and sex-matched controls were interviewed and asked the same questions as the cancer patients. Patients differed significantly from controls in that they had higher consumption of meats, cereals, total fats, total residue, and total fiber. They had also more previous other nonmalignant chronic diseases of the large bowel, and more direct relatives with cancer, mainly of the large bowel. They had also more professionals and more heavy smokers of cigarettes.

INTRODUCTION

The incidence of Cancer of the Large Bowel in Puerto Rico is among the lowest in the world (De Jong, 1972; Doll, 1970, 1966; Martínez, 1975; Roger, 1977). However, this low incidence has increased significantly during the last two decades (Martínez, 1967, 1975). These recent changes justified the exploration of factors associated with this disease in Puerto Rico. Because of the relative isolation of the population and the reliable population-based Central Cancer Registry data collected from all hospitals, pathology laboratories and through systematic search for cancer cases in the Island, this case-control study was made. This study reports on patients obtained with a diagnosis of adenocarcinoma of the large bowel in Puerto Rico between January 1, 1973 and February 28, 1975. It explores differences between cases and controls in relation to environmental factors, diet, previous large-bowel diseases, and familial aggregation. The hypothesis to be tested was: adenocarcinomas of the colon and rectum are more frequently diagnosed among patients with a diet high in meat and fat but low in fiber, abnormal bowel habits, other previous large bowel diseases, and familial aggregation of cancer; than a similar group of the population without these characteristics (controls).

45

MATERIALS AND METHODS

The study was designed to interview patients with a histologic diagnosis of adenocarcinoma of the large bowel and a minimum of 20 years of residency in Puerto Rico.

The total number of cases diagnosed with adenocarcinoma of the large bowel in
Puerto Rico residents for the years 1973 and 1974 were 540. Some cases were obtained after the study was closed (late reports), and others were disclosed during
the interview that were not residents of Puerto Rico for 20 years. The Central
Cancer Registry has a systematic search of cancer cases, and we consider that for
this reason and for the number of late reports involved, the factors of the delay
and non residence are not related to the hypothesis to be tested.

During the 26-months period, 463 patients with adenocarcinomas of the colon and
rectum (rubrics 153 and 154 ICD, 8th Rev. WHO, 1968) in both sexes fulfilled the
requirements. Four hundred and sixty-one (461) were interviewed, and two refused.

For each cancer patient, one control without any reported malignancy was matched
by age (within 5 years) and sex. The control was selected from the same community
as the patient, and had lived there for at least 10 years. If the patient had died
or was incapable of answering the questions with apparent reliability, a member of
the family, who had lived for 10 years or more with the patient, was interviewed.
A similar interview was taken with his control, and the same person interviewed
each pair. From the 461 pairs, 102 had relatives interviewed.

Interviewers were trained specifically to obtain all answers of long-term dietary
and personal habits and so forth, for the period before the patient started with
symptoms of the disease. The questionnaire was tested in the field and modified
according to initial results.

The questionnaire included dietary questions in terms of frequency of consumption
per day, week, or month of foods usually eaten by cases and controls. Later in
the analysis, foods were assessed by their content of fat, total residue and fiber.[1]
There were also queries regarding bowel habits, stress, personal history of other
chronic previous diseases, and family history of malignant diseases. Lastly it
requested information of the usual social variables such as place of birth, usual
occupation, level of education, and use of tobacco and alcohol.

In the dietary history the frequency of consumption of each food was asked separately. No effort was made to quantify any food eaten by the persons involved in
the study (Hegsted, 1975). The material was analyzed with respect to: (a) Differences between cases and controls in the frequency of consumption of each common
type of food eaten in Puerto Rico, (b) Differences in the frequency of consumption
for each of three groups of foods: meats, cereals, and vegetables, and (c) Differences in the consumption of all foods weighting each food by its content of fats,
of total residue, and of fiber, in the usual portion separately (Church, 1970).
The frequency of consumption of each food was converted to yield the content of
each of the above; these "indexes" of consumption were classified as low, moderate,
and high.

Constipation was not asked as such; the questionnaire included instead a series of
15 questions as to frequency, consistency, and odor of stools; habitual place of
bowel movement (e.g. own house, office, anywhere); medicines and procedures taken
for defecation, etc. With the combination of the answers, the grade of chronic
constipation was determined and patients and controls classified into 3 categories:
high, low, and none.

The use of tobacco per day was investigated for cigarettes, cigars, pipes, and chewing tobacco. The duration of the habit was also recorded in years.

Familial aggregation of cancer was investigated for: (a) cancer of any primary site, (b) cancer of any organ of the digestive system, and (c) cancer of the large bowel. They were asked of in father, mother, and siblings; singly and in any possible combination of the three.

To determine differences between cases and controls, Mcnemar statistics was used for analysis of 2 categories and Fleiss and Everitt Chi square test for matched pairs when 3 categories were involved. The conventional method for calculating relative risk was used.

RESULTS

Location of Lesions

Of the 461 adenocarcinomas, 232 were in the colon (122 in males and 110 in females), and 229 in the rectum and rectosigmoid junction (131 in males and 98 in females). The overall male-female ratio was 1.2:1.

Background Information

Age - The age distribution of patients and controls was very similar between sexes. The highest percentage was in the group 65-74 years of age. Education and occupation - Almost fifteen percent of the patients but 10.4% of the controls had more than 12 years of school. The controls had 4% more illiterates than the cases. Twenty-two percent of the patients were professionals in contrast to 18.5% of the controls. In the total popualtion only 7.8% are estimated as professionals (Plan. Board Govern. P.R., 1977). Place of birth and residence -- Ninety-eight percent of the patients and 99.6% of the controls were born in Puerto Rico. Sixty five percent of the patients and 64% of the controls lived in metropolitan and urban areas of Puerto Rico for at least 20 years previous to the date of the interview. The estimate for the general urban population is 56% (Plan. Board Govern. P.R., 1977). Marital status - Among the cancer patients 34.9% were single, widowed, or divorced as compared with 34.1% of the controls. Religion - The great majority of Puerto Ricans are Catholics; nine patients and 6 controls belonged to the Seven Day Adventist sect and no Hebrews were found. Social stress - For the purpose of determining the effect of social stress on the physiology of the large bowel, eight different questions were included in the questionnaire but practically no differences were found between the two groups. Alcohol and tobacco - In the analysis of the usual types of alcoholic beverages patients always reported somewhat higher frequency than the controls, but the difference was not statistically significant. For each type of tobacco more patients than controls were heavy users, but the difference was significant only for cigarettes (29.1% heavy smokers among the patients vs 16.5% among the controls.)

Diet

Each food - We obtained the frequency of consumption of each common food eaten in Puerto Rico. Questions on the different types of meats were also asked in order to identify differences in specific consumption of beef. The patients reported significantly more frequent consumption than the controls only for the following individual foods: fatty cheeses, cottage cheese, eggs, ice cream, white bread, oatmeal, cream of wheat, and fruit juices.

Groups of foods - More patients than controls reported higher frequencies of consumption of all types of meats (34.7% vs 24.3%), and cereals (26.7% vs 18.7%).

The differences were significant at 0.001 level. The relative risk increased with the increasing consumption of these groups of foods. (Table 1)

TABLE 1 - Frequency of consumption of groups of foods by patients with adenocarcinomas of the large bowel and age- and sex matched controls. Puerto Rico, 1973-1974

Group of foods

	Cases	Controls	Total	R.R.
Meats				
Low	37	56	93	1.0
Medium	264	293	557	1.4
High	160	112	272	2.2
Total	461	461	922	x^2=16.5;P=<0.001
Cereals				
Low	23	51	74	1.0
Medium	315	323	638	2.2
High	123	87	210	3.1
	461	461	922	x^2=29.3;P=<0.001

Foods weighted by the amount of fat, total residue, and fiber - More patients than controls had higher consumption of fat (49.2% vs 36.7%), of total residue (36.4% vs 29.5%), and fiber (51.4% vs 42.3%). These differences are significant at 0.001 level for fat and 0.01 for total residue, but at 0.05 level for fiber. The relative risks increased with the increasing value of the indexes. The risk of a high consumption of fat is almost four times greater than for low consumption. (Table 2) In Puerto Rico the use of lard for cooking is still frequent, and the charcoal roasted pig is a meat frequently eaten in the Island.

TABLE 2 - Indexes of consumption for total fats, residue, and fiber in foods usually eaten by patients with adenocarcinoma of the large bowel, and age- and sex-matched controls. Puerto Rico 1973-1974

	Cases	Controls	Total	R.R.
FATS				
*Low	12	34	46	1.0
**Moderate	222	258	480	2.4
***High	227	169	396	3.8
Total	461	461	922	x^2=24.8P=<0.001
TOTAL RESIDUE				
*Low	20	45	65	1.0
**Moderate	273	280	553	4.9
***High	168	136	304	6.2
Total	461	461	922	x^2=14.8P=<0.01
FIBER				
*Low	33	41	74	1.0
**Moderate	191	225	416	1.1
***High	237	195	432	1.5
Total	461	461	922	x^2=8.3P=<0.05

Index is the sum for all foods of the frequency of consumption times the given weight, according with the content of the item in each food.

*Index Less than 150)		*Less than 200)	TOTAL	*Less than 90)	
**Index 150 - 224	) FATS	**200 - 299)	RESIDUE	**90 - 129)	FIBER
***Index 225 or more)		***300 or more)		***130 or more)	

Bowel habits - This analysis was made both with all cases and controls included (461 pairs), and with only those cases and controls personally interviewed (359 pairs), to explore possible differences in the responses of patients versus relatives. In both groups more patients than controls reported a higher grade of constipation. (Table 3)

TABLE 3 - Constipation of patients with adenocarcinomas of the large bowel and age and sex-matched controls. Puerto Rico 1973-74

	Cases	Controls	Total	R.R.
ALL PAIRS				
None*	331	402	733	1.0
Low**	119	54	173	2.7
High***	11	5	16	2.7
Total	461	461	922	

$$x^2=33.5 \quad P=< 0.001$$

	Cases	Controls	Total	R.R.
EXCLUDING RELATIVES' INTERVIEWS				
None*	185	268	453	1.0
Low**	135	76	211	2.6
High***	39	15	54	3.8
Total	359	359	718	

$$x^2=42.4 \quad P=< 0.001$$

*None less than 3 factors; **Low: 3 to 4 factors; ***High: 3 or more factors; Factors: Defecation every two weeks or more; Short or cibolous stools; Foul odor of stools; Hard consistency of stools; Great effort to defecate; Frequent tenesmus; Frequent mucous and/or bloody stools; Frequent use of laxatives and/or enemas and/or suppositories.

Previous diseases - During the years prior to diagnosis of the adenocarcinoma of the large bowel, significantly more cases than controls had suffered from the following diseases: Diverticulosis (8.0% vs 2.6%), Intestinal polyposis (4.6% vs 0.4%), Ulcerative colitis (3.5% vs 0.4%), other types of colitis (10.8% vs 3.3%), Chronic Constipation (39.0% vs 20.6%), Diarrheas (17.8% vs 8.6%), and Hemorrhoids (36.5% vs 16.4%). These differences are significant at 0.01 level. No significant differences were found for diseases such as: Schistosomiasis, intestinal tuberculosis, Crohn's disease, diabetes, obesity, and arterioesclerosis.

Family history of cancer - Patients always reported more direct relatives (father, mother, or siblings) with cancer than the controls for all cancer sites (103 vs 84) and for cancer of the digestive organs (39 vs 31), but it was only with respect to cancer of the large bowel where a significant difference was found at 0.05 level (22 relatives among the patients against 9 among the controls). (Table 4)

TABLE 4 - Familial aggregation of cancer of the large bowel in patients with adenocarcinomas of the large bowel and age-sex-matched controls. Puerto Rico, 1973-74

RELATIVES WITH CANCER	Cases	Controls	Total	
Father, mother & sibling	0	0	0	
Father & mother, no sibling	0	0	0	
Father or mother & sibling	2	0	2	
Father or mother or sibling	22	9	31	
None	437	452	889	$x^2=6.8; P < 0.05$
TOTAL	461	461	922	

I. Martinez *et al.*

DISCUSSION

The purpose of this case-control study was to explore the possible association of adenocarcinoma of the large bowel with the above mentioned factors. It was conducted having in mind the great limitations intrinsic in the interview method, such as the possible biases introduced by the memory factor, the inaccuracies of any long-term dietary history, the difficulties to confirm diagnosis of some past diseases, and the particular limitation of local scientific talent and technical resources to perform scientific work with modern sophisticated techniques.

There are controversial opinions as to the similarity of the adenocarcinomas diagnosed in the colon and those in the rectum. Unfortunately, resources available did not permit us to continue this study to obtain a large enough number of cases for breakdown by sub-sites and sex. For this reason the analysis was done with all locations of adenocarcinomas in the large bowel and sexes together as a group.

The diseases previous to the adenocarcinoma of the patients and the diseases of their relatives, were accepted at face value as reported by the cases and controls. In our media is very difficult to confirm such diagnoses. Experience tells us that: (a) many relatives of old patients are dead, (b) others do not remember where or by whom the disease was diagnosed, and (c) many do not permit the search for family pathology.

The use of tobacco and alcohol was asked solely as an indirect measure of social stress which in turn would affect colonic physiology and could contribute as co-factor in a complex causation. Although the association of the use of tobacco and carcinoma of the large intestine would not be incompatible the hypothesis of the ingestion with saliva of benzopyrenes or nitrosamines (Breslow, 1974; Roger, 1977).

The religion question was included for the purpose of exploring the number of patients and controls with special diets such as those of the Seven Day Adventists and Hebrews, as has been explored in other studies (Phillips, 1973).

In relation to the diet, it was considered from the initial planning of this study that no reliable quantification of the foods ingested would be obtained by questioning (Hegsted, 1975b). The most we can get with the interview method is frequency of the usual foods eaten. In spite of these deficiencies, we considered that in the population of this small Island the diet is quite uniform. To reduce some biases we also analyzed differences in groups of foods (meats, cereals, vegetables) and in a third step we designed three weighted indexes of consumption for the items under investigation (fats, residue, and fiber). This procedure refines somewhat the crudeness of just counting the frequency of each food, and also the frequencies of nonweighted groups of foods. Cancer cases reported higher frequencies of consumption of meats, cereals, total amount of fats, total residue, and fiber, than the controls. The inconsistent finding of patients and or their relatives reporting more constipation, but frequent consumption of some foods high in total residue including fiber may be a product of the recall biases expected in this type of study, or the difficulty in defining fiber (Hegsted, 1975a). However the strength of differences is much lower than differences for items like fats and meats.

The reported higher frequency of other previous large bowel chronic diseases in cancer patients than in the controls confirmed similar findings in other studies (Wynder, 1967). The higher frequency of cancer cases among direct relatives of the study cases (particularly in the large bowel), merits greater numbers of cases and more careful analysis from the genetic point of view.

The study agrees with some of the previously published data in terms of distribution of these tumors by socio-economic levels, occupation, etc. (Correa, 1966; Tannebaun, 1959; Wynder, 1967). It is also in agreement with the metabolic hypothesis which postulates that the higher the consumption of fats and meats, the higher the frequency of cancer of the large bowel (Haenszel, 1975; Tannebaun, 1959; Wynder, 1975). Our findings disagree in part with those who have found that diets high in fiber and residue are associated with a lower frequency of these tumors (Burkitt, 1971; Modan, 1975).

The higher consumption of meats, and foods with high content of fats, correlates with high socio-economic level. Both factors are the results of higher income (Correa, 1966).

The consumption of more expensive foods, such as meats and eggs, in Puerto Rico has changed during the last two decades. It parallels with the increasing of family income. More meats and more calories from fats should be expected, as it has occurred in the evolution of an almost completely agricultural country towards an industrialized one (Fernández, 1975; Martínez, 1966). Similar changes in frequency of food consumption have occurred among Puerto Ricans born and living in New York (Monk, 1975) and also in other ethnical groups with marked socio-economic changes (Haenszel, 1975; Tannebaun, 1959).

This study points out the need for continuation of research on the metabolism of fats and meats. (Wynder, 1975)

Future studies on time trends of the incidence of large bowel adenocarcinoma in Puerto Rico will elucidate whether the observed associations are maintained, and whether patterns of environmental and dietary habits undergoing change will result in alteration of the frequency of this disease in the Island.

REFERENCES

Church, Ch. F., and Church, H. N. (1970). Food Values of Portions Commonly Used. Philadelphia; J. B. Lippincott, Co., 11th Edition, 180.

Breslow, N.E. and Eustrom, J.E. (1974). Geographic correlation between cancer mortality rates and alcohol-tobacco consumption in United States. J. Natl. Cancer Institute, 53, 631-639.

Burkitt, D.P. (1971). Epidemiology of Cancer of the Colon and Rectum. Cancer, 28, 3-13.

Correa, P., and Llanos, G. (1966). Morbility and Mortality from Cancer in Cali, Colombia. J. Natl. Cancer Institute, 36, 717-745.

De Jong, V.W. et al. (1972). The Distribution of Cancer within the Large Bowel. Int. J. Cancer, 10, 463-477.

Doll, R., Muir, C., and Waterhouse, J. (Eds.) (1970). Cancer in Five Continents, Vol. II. Geneva: Union Internationale Contre le Cancer.

Doll, R., Payne, P., and Waterhouse, J. (Eds.) (1966). Cancer in Five Continents, Vol. I. Geneva: Union Internationale Contre le Cancer.

Fernández, N.A. (1975). Nutrition in Puerto Rico. Cancer Res., 35, 3272-3291.

Haenszel, W., Correa, P., and Cuello, C. (1975). Social Class Differences among Patients with Large-Bowel Cancer in Cali. J. Natl. Cancer Institute, 54, 1031-1035.

Haenszel, W., Berg, J.W., Sigi, M., et al. (1973). Large Bowel Cancer in Hawaiian Japanese. J. Natl. Cancer Institute, 51, 1765-1779.

Hegsted, D.M., in Scheniderman, M.A. (1975a). Summary of the Informal Discussion of Dietary Factors and Special Epidemiological Situations. Cancer Res.,35, 3540.

Hegsted, D.M. (1975b). Summary of the Conference on Nutrition in the Causation of Cancer. Cancer Res., 35, 3541-3543.

Martínez, I., Torres, R., and Frías, Z. (1975). Cancer Incidence in the Unites States and Puerto Rico. Cancer Res., 35, 3265-3271.

Martínez, I. (ed.) (1967). Cancer in Puerto Rico 1950-64. Puerto Rico: Central Cancer Registry, Div. of Cancer Control, Department of Health, Puerto Rico.

Martínez, I. (Ed.) (1965 to 1975). Cancer in Puerto Rico (Yearly reports), Puerto Rico: Central Cancer Registry, Div. of Ca. Control, Department of Health, Santurce, Puerto Rico.

Martínez, I. (1966). Factors Associated with Cancer of the Esophagus, Mouth, and Pharynx in Puerto Rico. J. Natl. Cancer Institute, 42:6, 1069-1094.

Modan, B., Barell, V., Lubin, F., and Modan, M. (1975). Dietary Factors and Cancer in Israel. Cancer Res., 35, 3503-3506.

Monk, M. and Warshaurer, M.E. (1975). Stomach and Colon Cancer Mortality among Puerto Ricans in New York City and Puerto Rico. J. Chrn. Dis., 28, 349-358.

Phillips, R.L., Kuzma, J.W., Lemon, F.R., et al. (1973). Mortality from colon-rectal cancer among California Seven-Day Adventists. Annual meeting of the A.P.H.A. San Francisco.

Planning Board Government of Puerto Rico (1977). Personal Communication.

Roger, W.R., and Horm, J.W. (1977). Association of Cancer Sites with Tobacco and Alcohol Consumption and Socio-economic Status of Patients. Interview Study from the Third National Cancer Survey. J. Natl. Cancer Institute, 58, 525-547.

Tannebaun, A. (1959). Nutrition and Cancer. In: F. Homberger (Ed.): Physiopathology of Cancer, New York: Hoeber-Harper, (Ed.) 2, 517-562.

Waterhouse, J., Muir, C., Correa, P., Powell, J., and Davis, W., (Eds.) (1976) Cancer in Five Continents, Vol. III. Lyon: A Technical Report of the I.A.R.C. Scientific Pub. No. 15.

Wynder, E.L. and Shigematsu, T. (1967). Environmental Factors of Cancer of the Colon and Rectum. Cancer, 20, 1520-1561.

Wynder, E.L., Hoffman, D., Chau, P. et al. (1975). Interdisciplinary and Experimental Approaches: Metabolic Epidemiology. In: Fraumeni, J.F., Editors. Persons at High Risk of Cancer. Academic Press, Inc. New York, 485.

The Role of Metabolic Epidemiology and Laboratory Studies in the Etiology of Colon Cancer

Gary M. Williams, Bandaru S. Reddy and John H. Weisburger

Naylor Dana Institute, American Health Foundation, 1 Dana Road, Valhalla, New York 10595, U.S.A.

ABSTRACT

Epidemiologic data on colon cancer incidence suggest a relationship to diet. Metabolic epidemiology and laboratory studies reveal that diet could be a source of carcinogens and probably contributes to colon cancer development through alteration of luminal constituents that act as tumor promotors. The dietary elements involved in the etiology of colon cancer appear to be high protein, high fat and low fiber.

INTRODUCTION

The geographic distribution of colon cancer shows the highest incidence rates in Western Europe and Anglo-Saxon countries, intermediate rates in Eastern Europe and the lowest rates in Africa, Asia and Latin America (Weisburger Reddy and Joftes, 1978). Evidence that this distribution is determined by environmental factors rather than genetic is provided by studies of migrants from regions of low risk to those of high risk (Buell and Dunn, 1965; Staszewski and Haenszel 1965). Based on these and other data, it has been proposed that colon cancer incidence is related to diet (Wynder, 1967, 1969; Burkitt, 1971; Armstrong and Doll, 1975). Subsequent descriptive epidemiologic studies have in large measure confirmed the role of diet with some noteable exceptions (Enstrom, 1975). However, such studies have not lead to the recognition of the possibly multifactorial causes and determinants involved in this disease. Therefore, the elucidation of this complex problem is being pursued in our Institute by a multidisciplinary effort. Metabolic epidemiology and laboratory studies have lead to important insights into the role of dietary consitituents.

Fat

Wynder and coworkers (1969) first proposed that colon cancer incidence is mainly associated with dietary fat. Hill and co-workers (1971) demonstrated a correlation between the fecal concentration of steroids and the incidence of colon cancer in 6 countries. It was subsequently shown that fecal excretion of cholesterol metabolites, coprostanol and coprostanone, and bile acids was higher in groups of populations consuming a high fat, mixed-Western diet than in groups consuming diets low in fat (Reddy and Wynder, 1973) (Table 1).

Table 1. Daily fecal neutral sterol and bile acid excretion in different populations

Population groups	Total bile acids[a] (mg/day)	Total neutral sterols[b] (mg/day)
Americans (17)[c]	256 + 34[d,e]	817 + 115[e]
American vegetarian (12)	133 + 15	318 + 53
American Seventh-Day Adventists (11)	54 + 16	266 + 42
Japanese (18)	83 + 8	266 + 29
Chinese (11)	54 + 13	195 + 38

a - includes cholic, deoxycholic, lithocholic, and other bile acids.
b - includes cholesterol, coprostanol and coprostanone
c - number of subjects are shown in parentheses.
d - Mean + SE
e - Significantly different from other population groups

Furthermore the fecal bile acid concentration was found to be higher in colon cancer patients than controls (Reddy and Wynder, 1977).

In model studies in rats, those consuming a high fat diet were more susceptible to colon tumor induction by a variety of carcinogens than animals on a low fat regimen (Nigro and coworkers, 1975; Reddy, Watanabe and Weisburger, 1977) (Table 2).

Table 2. Intestinal tumor incidence induced by carcinogens
          in F344 rats fed low or high fat diets[a]

| Carcinogen | Diet % beef fat | Animals with intestinal tumors | |
		Small intestine %	Colon %
1,2-dimethylhydrazine	5	20	23
	20	13	60
methylazoxymethanol acetate	5	7	40
	20	13	67
methylnitrosourea	5	0	23
	20	0	73

[a] from Reddy, Watanabe and Weisburger (1977).

Rats on a high-fat diet, just as humans, excreted more fecal bile acids and steroid metabolites (Reddy and coworkers, 1977).

The role of bile acids identified in the metabolic epidemiologic studies was supported by the findings of Nigro and associates (1973, 1974) that procedures leading to increased bile acid excretion would enhance the development of tumors initiated by chemical carcinogens. The evidence of the importance of bile acids as colon tumor promotors came from studies by Narisawa and coworkers (1974) and Reddy and coworkers (1976, 1977). In these studies individual bile acids were shown to exert a promoting effect on the development of colon tumors induced in rats by chemical carcinogens (Table 3). Secondary bile acids were somewhat more effective than primary bile acids.

Table 3. Promoting effect of bile acids on colorectal tumor
          induction by intrarectal N-methyl-N'-nitro-N-
          nitrosoguandidine (MNNG) in conventional and germfree
          F344 rats[a].

	Animals with tumors %	Total Tumors
Conventional		
MNNG[b]	25	10
MNNG & lithocholic acid	52	30
MNNG & taurodeoxycholic acid	62	28
lithocholic acid	0	0
taurodeoxycholic acid	0	0
Germfree		
MNNG	89	38
MNNG & deoxycholic acid	82	75
deoxycholic acid	0	0

[a] from Reddy, Weisburger and Wynder (1978)
[b] N-methyl-N'-nitro-N-nitrosoguandine.

Thus, our current hypothesis on the role of dietary fat in the
etiology of colon cancer is as follows: (a) compounds within the
colon with properites of carcinogens or of cocarcinogens and
promoters that would lead to the development of colon cancer, are
associated with dietary habits and (b) the high-fat diet changes
the concentration of secondary bile acids in the gut and also the
metabolic activity of gut bacteria which may produce tumorigenic
compounds from bile acids (these bile acids have been shown to
act as colon tumor promoters).

Fiber

The studies of Burkitt (1971, 1974) called attention to the
importance of lack of dietary fiber in the etiology of intestinal
disease, including colon cancer. Our recent investigations have
revealed a possible link between the protective effect of fiber
and the role of fat. For one thing diets high in fiber are
generally low in fat and thus would be protective for that reason.
However, even if the fat content remained constant, fiber by
increasing fecal bulk could lead to dilution of the promoting
bile acids. This concept appears to be sustained by recent
metabolic epidemiologic studies of groups at different risk. The
Finns have a low risk of colon cancer (Doll, 1969; Jensen and
coworkers, 1974) although they consume diets high in fat. The
explanation appears to relate to the high content of cereal fiber in
their diet, such that their fecal bulk is increased and their

fecal bile acid concentration reduced (Reddy and coworkers, 1978). However, the role of fiber may be more complex than simply providing fecal bulk since fibers are known to differ in their capacity to bind bile acids (Kritchevsky and Story, 1974). This possibility is sustained by ongoing laboratory studies in our Institute that show that addition of certain fibers such as pectin to the diet reduces the colon cancer incidence in experimental animals whereas others have no protective effect (Table 4). The mechanism may thus relate to bile acid binding rather than simple dilution. This phenomenon of different effects of various fibers may account for discrepancies in experimental findings on the protective effect of fiber (Ward, Yamamato and Weisburger, 1973; Freeman, Spiller and Kim, 1978).

Table 4.   Intestinal tumor incidence in F344 rats fed diets containing various fibers or tannic acid and treated with azoxymethane[a]

Diets	Animals with colon tumors %	Colon tumors per rat	Per tumor bearing rat
Control	57	0.8	1.5
Pectin	10	0.1	1.0
Alfalfa	53	0.7	1.3
Wheat bran	33	0.4	1.2
Tannic acid	30	0.3	1.1

[a] Watanabe and coworkers, in preparation

Protein

Protein has also been considered to be involved in colon cancer causation (Hill and Drasar, 1974). In a study which examined the effect of 7.5%, 15% and 22.5% dietary protein on colon carcinogenesis induced in rats by 1,2-dimethylhydrazine, the incidence was affected by the protein level, but the total number of tumors increased with protein level. An important lead on the role of protein discovered in the laboratory of Sugimura was that broiling of protein-containing foods yielded mutagens on the food surface (Nagao and coworkers, 1977). A decisive finding was that a product from the pyrolysis of tryptophan was a gamma-carboline derivative (Sugimura and coworkers, 1977; Nagao and coworkers, 1977) that was an o-methylarylamine type of compound. Conceptually, this is most intriguing since o-methylarylamines such as 2'3-dimethyl-4-aminobiphenyl usually induce colon cancer in male animals and breast and colon cancer in female animals (Weisburger 1979). This mutagen, abbreviated Trp-P-1 1 is also active in the hepatocyte primary culture/DNA

repair test developed in our laboratory (Williams, 1976; 1977)
(Table 5). It is being tested for carcinogenicity by Dr. Sugimura.

Table 5. Activity of TRP-1 in the hepatocyte primary culture/
DNA Repair Test[a]

| Compound | DNA Repair[b] | |
	Exp 1	Exp 2
Trp-P-1[c]	9.8	9.1
none	0.4	0.9

[a] performed according to Williams (1978)
[b] average grains/nucleus
[c] provided by Dr. T. Sugimura, National Cancer Center, Tokyo

Bruce and coworkers (1977) reported that mutagens are present in
the feces of humans and this finding has been confirmed by Reddy
and associates at this Institute. Of 47 samples tested thus far 25
have been positive in the Ames test (Table 6).

Table 6   Fecal Mutagenic Activity of Healthy Controls Consuming a
mixed-western Diet[a]

| | Without Microsomal Activation | | | With Microsomal Activation | | |
	TA100	TA98	Both	TA100	TA98	Both
No. of Samples Positive (Total 25)	13	18	7	3	2	1

[a] Unpublished observations, Reddy and coworkers 1977.

The amount of Fecal mutagen can be reduced by administering vitamin
(Bruce and coworkers, 1977) suggesting that some might arise from
nitrosation of dietary amines.

The nature of these fecal mutagens is of considerable importance
because they may represent the carcinogenic principles that
initiate the malignant conversion of colon cells. The subsequent
fate of "initiated" cells would then be highly dependent upon the

modulating influence of other dietary factors such as bile acids
and fiber.

Conclusion

Descriptive epidemiologic investigations have led to the recognition
of the importance of diet in the development of colon cancer.
Further understanding of this relationship must now be pursued by
multidisciplinary approaches involving metabolic epidemiology and
laboratory studies. Such approaches are yielding a mechanistic
explanation of the role of specific dietary consitituents in the
etiology of this disease and thus will provide the scientific base
for the institution of rational preventive measures.

REFERENCES

Armstrong B and R. Doll (1975) Environmental factors and the
    incidence and mortality from cancer in different countries with
    special reference to dietary practices. Int. J. Cancer. 15:
    617.
Berg, J.W. (1977). World-wide variations in cancer incidence as
    clues to cancer origins. In. Origins of Human Cancer. Cold
    Spring Harbor Laboratory. pp15.
Bruce, W.R. and coworkers (1977). A mutagen in the feces of normal
    humans. In Origins of Human Cancer. Cold Spring Harbor
    Laboratory New York. pp1641-1642.
Buell, P., and J.E. Dunn. (1965). Cancer mortality among Japanese
    Issei and Nisei of California. Cancer 18. 656.
Burkitt, D.P. (1971). Epidemiology of cancer of the colon and rectum.
    Cancer 28. 3.
Burkitt, D.P. (1974). An epidemiological approach to cancer of the
    large intestine. Dis. Colon Rectum. 17. 456.
Chomchai, C. N. Bhadrachari, and N. D. Nigro. (1974). The effect
    of bile on the induction of experimental intestinal tumours in
    rats. Dis. Colon Rectum. 17. 310.
Correa, P. and W. Haenszel (1978). The epidemiology of large-bowel
    cancer. Advances in Cancer Research 26. 2-141.
Doll, R. (1969). The geographic distribution of cancer.
    Br. J. Cancer 23. 1-8.
Enstrom, J.E. (1975) Colorectal cancer and consumption of beef and
    fat. Brit J. Cancer. 32. 432-439.
Freeman, H.J. G.A. Spiller and Y.S.Kim (1978) A double-blind
    study on 1,2-dimethylhydrazine-induced rat colonic
    neoplasm Cancer Res. 38. 2912-2917.
Hill, M.J. and coworkers (1971) Bacteria and aetiology of cancer
    of the large bowel. Lancet i 95.
Jensen, O.M., and coworkers (1974). A comparative study of
    the diagnositc basis for cancer of the colon and
    cancer of the rectum in Denmark and Finland.
    Int. J. Epidemiol 3. 183-186.
Kritchevsky D. and J.A. Story. (1974). Binding of bile salts in
    vitro by non-nutritive fiber. J. Nutr. 104. 458-462.

60   G. M. Williams, B. S. Reddy and J. H. Weisburger

Nagao, M. and coworkers (1977). Mutagenicities of smoke condensates and the charred surface of fish and meat. Cancer Letters 2. 221-226.

Narisawa, T. and coworkers. (1974). Promoting effect of bile acids on colon carcinogenesis after intrarectal instillation of N-Methyl-N'-nitro-N-nitrosoguanidine in rats. J. Natl. Cancer Inst. 53. 1093-1097.

Nigro, N.D. and coworkers (1975). Effect of dietary beef fat on intestinal tumor formation by azoxymethane in rats. J. Natl. Cancer Inst. 54. 429-442.

Reddy, B.S. and Wynder, E.L. (1973). Large bowel carcinogenesis. Fecal constituents of populations with diverse incidence rates of colon cancer. J. Natl. Cancer Inst. 50. 1437-1442.

Reddy, B.S. and coworkers (1976) Promoting effect of sodium deoxycholate on adenocarcinomas in germfree rats. J. Natl. Cancer Inst. 56. 441-442.

Reddy, B.S. and coworkers (1977). Promoting effect of bile acids in colon carcinogenesis in germ-free and conventional F344 rats. Cancer Res. 37. 3238.

Reddy, B.S. K. Watanabe and J.H. Weisburger (1977). Effect of high-fat diet on colon carcinogenesis in F344 rats treated with 1,2-dimethylhydrazine, methlazoxymethanol acetate or methylnitrosourea. Cancer Res. 37. 4156-4159.

Reddy and coworkers (1977) Effect of type and amount of dietary fat and 1,2-dimethylhydrazine on biliary bile acids, fecal bile acids and neutral sterols in rats. Cancer Res. 37. 2132-2137.

Reddy, B.S. J.H. Weisburger and E.L. Wynder (1978) Colon Cancer. Bile salts as tumor promoters. In T.J. Slaga, A. Sivak and R.K. Boutwell (Ed) Carcinogenesis 2. Mechanisms of Tumor Promotion and Cocarcinogenesis 453-464

Reddy, B.S. and coworkers. (1978) Fecal constituents of a high-risk Finnish population for the development of large bowel cancer. Cancer Letters 4. 217-222.

Sugimura, T. and coworkers (1977). Mutagenic principle(s) in tryptophan and phenylalanine pyrolysis products. Proc. Japan Acad 53. 58-61.

Seino, Y. and coworkers. (1977). Mutagen-carcinogens in food, with special reference to highly mutagenic pyrolytic products in broiled foods. In Origins of Human Cancer, Cold Spring Harbor Laboratory, New York.pp1561.

Topping D.C. and W.J. Visek (1976) Nitrogen intake and tumorigenesis in rats injected with 1,2-dimethylhydrazine. J. Nutri 106. 1583-1590.

Ward, J.M. R.S. Yamamoto and J.H. Weisburger (1973). Cellulose dietary bulk and azoxymethane-induced intestinal cancer. J. Natl. Cancer Inst. 51: 713-715.

Weisburger, J.H. and G.M. Williams (1979). Chemical Carcinogenesis In. James F. Holland and Emil Frei III (Ed.) Cancer Medicine Lea & Febinger, Philadelphia.

Weisburger J.H. (1979) Mechanism of action of diet as a carcinogen, Cancer in press.

Weisburger J.H., B.S. Reddy and D.L. Joftes (1975) Colo-Rectal Cancer UICC Technical Report Series 19 1-143.

Williams, G.M. (1976) Carcinogen-induced DNA repair in primary rat
    liver cell cultures; a possible screen for chemical
    carcinogens. Cancer Letters 1. 231-236.
Williams, G.M. (1977) The detection of chemical carcinogens by
    unscheduled DNA synthesis in rat liver primary cell cultures
    Cancer Res. 37 1845-1851.
Wynder, E.L. and T. Shigematsu. (1967) Environmental factors of
    cancer of the colon and rectum. Cancer 20. 1520.
Wynder, E.L. and coworkers (1969). Environmental factors of cancer
    of the colon and rectum. II. Japanese epidemiological data.
    Cancer 23. 1210.

Epidemiology of Precancerous Lesions of the Gastrointestinal Tract in Sao Paulo, Brazil

C. Marigo

Departamento de Patologia, Faculdade de Ciências Médicas de Santa Casa,
Rua Cesário Motta Jr., 112 - CEP 01221, Sao Paulo, Brazil

ABSTRACT

All material of this study has been provided by gross and microscopic examination of surgical and necropsy specimens from a general hospital and Coroner Office. Dysplasia, carcinoma in situ and invasive carcinoma of esophagus occur frequently in the same specimen suggesting common epidemiological implications. Intestinal metaplasia of gastric mucosa is more severe in men going along with the two fold incidence of cancer in men compared with women; migrants from rural areas show higher prevalence than natives, probably by action of agents early in life. Data on adenomatous polyp and cancer of bowel show São Paulo as a community in a transitional stage from intermediate to high risk of cancer; migrants living for many years in São Paulo show same prevalence of natives suggesting action of agents in late decades; black natives have higher prevalence than African's; diverticula, hemorrhoid and appendicitis are positively associated with adenomatous polyp; these four lesions are negatively associated with lymphoid hyperplasia, suggesting immunological implications; adenomatous polyp is not related to schistosomiasis and do not appear to be precursor of low rectum cancer.

— Precancerous lesions; epidemiology; dysplasia; esophagus; intestinal metaplasia; stomach; adenomatous polyps; colon; rectum.

INTRODUCTION

The prevalence of precancerous and precursor lesions of gastointestinal tract in several countries at varying risk to cancer has been described to investigate their role in the genesis of cancer. Studies on epithelial dysplasia of esophagus (Mukada, Sato and Sasano, 1976), intestinal metaplasia of gastric mucosa (Morson, 1955; Stemmermann and Hayashi, 1968; Correa, Cuello and Duque, 1970; Salas, 1977) and adenomatous polyps of colon and rectum (Morson, 1962; Correa and co-workers, 1972; Stemmermann and Yatani, 1973; Sato and co-workers, 1976; Correa and co-workers, 1977) provide data on geographic pathology.

Similar study emphasizing epidemiologic characteristics has been carried out in the city of São Paulo in southeast of Brazil, where the incidence of cancer of those organs is intermediate in the international scale (Waterhouse and co-workers, 1976).

MATERIAL AND METHODS

Surgical material was obtained only from Hospital Central da Santa Casa de São Paulo, while necropsy material originate also from Coroner Office. All gross and microscopic procedures was performed in the years 1973 - 1978.

A systematic search for dysplasia and carcinoma in situ of the epithelial membrane of esophagus was done in a preliminary study of 30 surgical specimens of carcinoma by gross and microscopic examination of the whole mucosa.

The search for intestinal metaplasia of gastric mucosa was done in 79 surgical specimens of carcinoma following the same method of esophagus and in 760 autopsy specimens free of cancer following published gross and microscopic procedures (Correa and co-workers, 1970). Another series of 199 cancer cases of the register was analised to correlate with intestinal metaplasia in migrant populations.

832 specimens of large bowel from necropsies were used to search adenomatous polyps and other lesions following published gross and microscopic procedures (Correa and co-workers, 1972). Correlation of all lesions with carcinoma was made analising 407 cases of cancer from the register.

Data on sex, age, race and place of birth obtained were analised following several statistical procedures.

RESULTS AND DISCUSSION

ESOPHAGUS

In our series of 30 surgical specimens a total of 20 (66.6%) showed dysplasia and / or in situ carcinoma in the transitional area between normal epithelial and invasive carcinoma.   40% (12 / 30) showed dysplasia, 46.6% (14 / 30) in situ carcinoma and 20% (6 / 30) both lesions in the same specimen. Recent study in Japan (Mukada and co-workers, 1976) using esophagus of autopsies from four prefectures showed 36.7% of dysplasia and conclude that, irrespective of population risk of carcinoma, environmental factors inducing dysplasia of the esophageal epithelium exist universally and suggest the possibility of dysplasia develop under conditions of long-standing irritation. The higher incidence of in situ carcinoma in our series of surgical specimens, when compared with necropsy series of Japan, suggests that those factors induce the sequence dysplasia - in situ carcinoma - invasive carcinoma.

STOMACH

Surgical specimens of cancer showed 82% of intestinal metaplasia of gastric mucosa (Okuyama and Marigo, unpublished data). Necropsy series (Okuyama, 1977) showed a frequency of 50% in the age group over 30 years. These data place São Paulo in an intermediate position between countries with low and high incidence. There is not sex differences in prevalence, however in man the lesions are more extensive and severe, probably reflecting the male / female 2:1 ratio of gastric cancer mortality. Observed cases of intestinal metaplasia and cancer among migrants from rural areas, namely Minas Gerais State in southeast and Bahia State in northeast are significantly higher than expected when specific populations living in São Paulo are used for calculation. São Paulo natives show a inverse situation (Table 1).

TABLE 1   Observed (0) and Expected * (E) Cases of Gastric Cancer and Intestinal Metaplasia of Gastric Mucosa by Place of Birth

	Cancer		Intestinal Metaplasia	
	0	E	0	E
São Paulo City	90	150	106	203
Minas Gerais State	38	17	53	23
Bahia State	28	10	35	19

* Calculated using specif populations living in São Paulo.

This probably means that the factors affecting risk are common for both lesions and begin its action in the place of birth and early in life, as had been suggested by others (Correa and co-workers, 1970; Haenszel, 1975).

COLON AND RECTUM

The studies of necropsy and surgical specimens supplied the following informations (Marigo, Correa and Haenszel, 1978): sex differences in prevalence are minimal for cancer and adenomatous polyps. Polyp formation may be a function of surface area at risk, the greatest intestine lenght showing the higher polyp prevalence. Blacks of Brazil acquired the intermediate risk of white population for adenomatous polyps when compared with African experience. Migrants from Northeast of Brazil under 60 years of age have a low frequency of polyps and diverticula while after 60 the frequency approaches that of São Paulo natives (Table 2), probably due to exposition to local environmental factors prior to dead for many years.

TABLE 2   Age-Specific Prevalence (per 100 specimens) of Adenomatous Polyps and Diverticula by Place of Birth. São Paulo, 1973 - 1975.

	Number of Specimens	With Adenomatous Polyps	Diverticula
		%	%
São Paulo City			
0 — 29	143	2.1	—
30 — 59	139	14.4	10.1
60 +	94	25.5	20.2
Northeast of Brazil			
0 — 29	61	3.3	—
30 — 59	68	4.1	3.1
60 +	64	23.4	18.8
Minas Gerais			
0 — 29	32	6.3	—
30 — 59	71	14.1	8.5
60 +	43	30.2	11.6
Foreign-born			
30 — 59	12	16.7	16.7
60 +	29	55.2	24.1

There is a positive association in the distribution of adenomatous polyps, diverticulosis and hemorrhoid which tend to cluster in the same individuals, going along with Burkitt (1969, 1971) suggestion of some influence of diet in western communities at high risk of colon cancer. Lymphoid hyperplasia is negatively associated with adenomatous polyp, appendectomy, appendicitis, diverticulosis and hemorrhoid (odds ratio respectively of 0,15; 0,17; 0,14; 0,10; 0,10), suggesting a relation between adenomatous polyp prevalence and the immunologic status of the host. Schistosomiasis is not related to adenomatous polyp. Epidemiologic characteristics of low rectum cancer are unrelated to colon cancer and adenomatous polyp do not appear to be a precursor of low-rectum cancer (distribution of colorectal adenomatous polyps according to location shows for mid and low rectum only 3,5% in males and 9,18% in female, beeing these figures for colorectal cancer respectively of 50.5% and 42.1%).

The informations presented here and in related publications allow us to postulate that in near future the epidemiology of precursor lesions of gastrointestinal tract shall be one of the best sources for clues to prevent the majority of gastrointestinal cancer. Therefore, all kind of research on this field must be encouraged.

REFERENCES

Burkitt, D.P. (1969).   Related disease — related cause? Lancet, 2, 1229—1231.
Burkitt, D.P. (1971).   Epidemiology of Cancer of the Colon and rectum. Cancer, 28, 3—13
Correa, P., Cuello, C. and E. Duque (1970).   Carcinoma and intestinal metaplasia of the stomach in Colombian migrants. J. Natl. Cancer Inst., 44, 297—306.
Correa, P., Duque, E., Cuello, C. and W. Haenszel (1972).   Polyps of colon and rectum in Cali, Colombia. Int. J. Cancer, 9, 86—96.
Correa, P., Strong, J.P., Reif, A. and W. D. Johnson (1977).   The epidemiology of colorectal polyps. Prevalence in New Orleans and international comparison. Cancer, 39, 2258—2264.
Haenszel, W. (1975).   Migrant studies. In J. F. Fraumeni Jr. (Ed.), Persons at high risk of cancer. An approach to cancer etiology and control. Academic Press, New York, pp. 361—371.
Marigo, C., Correa, P. and W. Haenszel (1978).   Cancer and 'cancer related' colorectal lesions in São Paulo, Brazil. To be published in Int. J. Cancer, December.
Morson, B.C. (1955).   Intestinal metaplasia of the gastric mucosa. Br. J. Cancer, 9, 365—376.
Morson, B.C. (1962).   Some peculiarities in the histology of intestinal polyps. Dis. Colon Rectum, 5, 337—344.
Mukada, T., Sato, E. and N. Sasano (1976).   Comparative studies on dysplasia of esophageal epithelium in four prefectures of Japan (Miyagi, Nara, Wakayama and Aomori) with reference to risk of carcinoma. Tohoku J. exp. Med., 119, 51—63.
Okuyama, M.H. (1977).   Contribuição ao estudo da "metaplasia intestinal" na mucosa gástrica na cidade de São Paulo. Thesis presented at Faculdade de Ciências Médicas da Santa Casa de São Paulo, Brazil.
Sato, E., Ouchi, A., Sasano, N. and T. Ishidate (1976).   Polyps and diverticulosis of large bowel in autopsy population of Akita prefecture, compared with Miyagi. Cancer, 37, 1316—1321.
Stemmerman, G.N. and T. Hayashi (1968).   Intestinal metaplasia of gastric mucosa: a gross microscopic study of its distribution in various disease states. J. Natl. Cancer Inst., 41, 627—638.
Stemmerman, G.N. and R. Yatani (1973).   Diverticulosis and polyps of the large intestine. A necropsy study of Hawaii Japanese. Cancer, 31, 1260—1270.
Waterhouse, J., Muir, C., Correa, P. and J. Powell (1976).   Cancer incidence in five continents, Vol. III. IARC Scientific Publications No. 15, International Agency for Research on Cancer, Lyon.

Precancerous Lesions of the Alimentary Tract in Relation to Some Epidemiological Data in Japan

E. Sato*, M. Tokunaga* and T. Ishidate**

*Second Department of Pathology, Kagoshima University, Kagoshima, Japan
**First Department of Pathology, Akita University, Akita, Japan

ABSTRACT

A necropsy study of polypoid lesions of the large bowel in the Japanese prefectures of Akita and Miyagi indicated that adenomas in the high risk population for colo-rectal carcinoma (Akita) showed more frequent incidence and more severe atypia than those in Miyagi, an average risk. The measurement of nuclear DNA in adenoma cells revealed that an increased number of cells with large amount of DNA tend to appear with the advance of the degree of atypia. Epithelial dysplasia of the esophagus is not always related to the death rates for esophageal carcinoma in several prefectures. However, in the prefecture with the highest risk, the preva-lence of an advanced degree of dysplasia seemed to be related to epidemiological data. In the measurement of nuclear DNA contant, severe dysplasia showed a strong resemblance to the distribution pattern of high ploidy cells in esophageal carcino-ma. A comparative study on the degree of intestinalization of the stomach as re-vealed by alkaline phosphatase activity in surgical specimens showed that high risk population for gastric carcinoma (Akita) had a stomach mucosa with more severe and extensive intestinalization than the low risk population (Kagoshima) in Japan.

INTRODUCTION

Epithelial dysplasia of the esophagus, intestinalization of the stomach and adeno-matous polyps of the large intestine are thought to be major precancerous lesions of the alimentary tract. In Japan, carcinomas of the esophagus and of the stomach are very prevalent but the incidence of the cancer of the large bowel is not as high as in other western countries. However,the mortality rates for these cancers are extremely variable among the 47 prefectures in Japan, according to the epide-miological analysis by Segi (1974). In connection with the epidemiological data, necropsy studies on the degree, distribution and incidence of epithelial dysplasia of the esophagus and polypoid lesions of the large bowel have been performed on some selected subjects in high and low risk areas of Japan. In addition, a com-parative study has been made of the severity of intestinalization of the stomach as grossly revealed by alkaline phosphatase reaction on surgical specimens from two prefectures, one with a high and one with a low death rates, for gastric carcinoma.

RESULTS

Epithelial Dysplasia of the Esophagus

A total of 434 esophagi with no grossly detectable carcinoma were collected from
6 prefectures. The examination on subserial sections revealed that dysplasia was
found in 200 (46.1 %) cases, of which 70 had moderate and severe degree (higher
degrees). As shown in Table 1, the incidence of these higher degrees appeared not
to be related to the prevalence of the prefectural death rate for esophageal carcinoma except for one prefecture with the highest risk where men habitually drink
liquor named Shochu, stronger than rice wine (Sake);the latter is a common drink
throughout Japan. There was an apparent male preponderance in the incidenc of the
higher degrees of dysplasia in this prefecture,and the result corresponded with
the death rate data.
Then we measured the nuclear DNA content in dysplastic cells and in carcinoma cells
of the esophagus. As indicated in Table 2 it is obvious that the more histological
atypia of dysplasia advances, the more the amount of nuclear DNA increases,thus
there is strong resemblance of the DNA content of severe dysplasia and carcinoma
cells.

Table 1. Death Rate for Esophageal Cancer and Prevalence
of Dysplasia

Prefecture	Death rates		Advanced degree of dysplasia	
	Male	Female	Male	Female
Aomori	17.6 (35)*	4.4 (44)*	13.6%	5.6%
Akita	26.8 (17)	4.7 (37)	26.5	14.0
Miyagi	33.8 (3)	11.6 (3)	8.7	18.4
Nara	29.2 (12)	15.1 (1)	8.3	18.6
Wakayama	34.9 (2)	14.8 (2)	12.1	0
Kagoshima	37.2 (1)	8.4 (10)	36.2	7.8

* Figures in parentheses indicate the order of frequency in
46 prefectures

Table 2. Nuclear DNA Content in Normal,Dysplastic and Carcinoma
Cells

	DNA Content,percent			
	2c	4c	6c	8c-
Normal	91%	9%	-	-
Dysplasia				
Mild	81.2	18.3	0.5	-
Moderate	77.5	21.5	1	-
Severe	35	53.7	10.3	1
Carcinoma	47.3	39.5	11	2.2

Adenomas of the Large Bowel

Prevalence and histologic features of adenomatous polyps were examined on the
necropsy materials from two prefectures,Akita and Miyagi, using an illuminating
magnifying lens. According to Segi's analysis (1974) of mortality rates for colorectal carcinoma in individual prefectures of Japan, that of Akita is highest and
of Miyagi average. A total of 771 intestines were examined, of these 471 were
from Miyagi and 300 from Akita. Adenomas of the large bowel were more numerous
in Akita (30 %) than in Miyagi (18.3 %). When the materials were limited to these
over 20 years of age, Akita showed 37.9 % (64 positive cases among 169 intestines)

for males and 23.6 % (26 among 110) for females,while Miyagi had 27.5 % (65 among 236) for males and 18.0 % (24 among 133) for females. Furthermore, adenomas in Akita revealed more advanced structural and cytological atypia than those in Miyagi (Table 3).

Table 3. Degree of Histologic Atypia in Adenomas with Diameter of 5 - 9.9 mm

	Structural atypia			Cytological atypia			
	Mild	Moderate	Severe	0	I	II	III
Akita	21 (47)	22 (49)	2 (4)	25 (56)	13 (29)	5 (11)	2 (4)
Miyagi	14 (56)	11 (44)	0 0	14 (56)	10 (40)	1 (4)	0 0

Percent in parentheses

In the measurement of nuclear DNA content of adenoma cells with several degrees of histological atypia, histograms of adenoma indicate that an increased number of high content DNA nuclei tend to appear with the advance of the degree of atypia; the mode values shift to an area of near tetraploidy (Fig. la). Some adenomas showed a similar histogram pattern to that of carcinoma cells (Fig. lb).

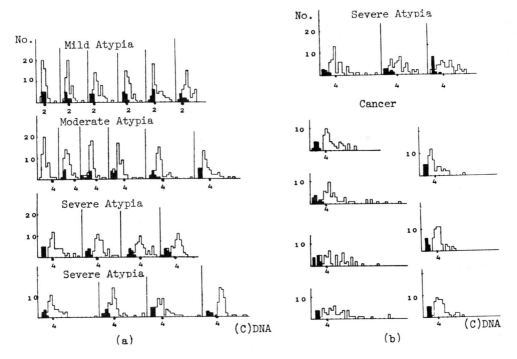

Fig. 1   Histogram of nuclear DNA content in adenomas with several grades of histological atypia(a),and in adenoma with severe atypia and carcinoma of the large bowel(b)

Intestinalization of Stomach

The intensity and extent of intestinalization of the stomach were compared in the surgical materials from Akita and Kagoshima Prefecture, using a method of grossly visible reaction of alkaline phosphatase activity as an indicator for the lesion. According to epidemiological data Akita is conspicuously prevalent for gastric carcinoma, whereas Kagoshima has the lowest level for the cancer in Japan. Table 4 shows that in carcinoma cases the mucosa tends to have strong intestinalization in both prefectures, although the Akita cases are more advanced than the cases from Kagoshima, especially in the younger generation. However, in the benign cases the degree of intestinalization is quite different; Akita cases are far more severe than Kagoshima. The result indicates that there is a high incidence and an advanced degree of intestinalization in a high risk population for gastric cancer, even if the people do not have a cancer.

Table 4. Age and Grade of Intestinalization in Stomach Carcinoma and Ulcer Cases

Intestinalization

Age		Carcinoma						Ulcer					
		Akita			Kagoshima			Akita			Kagoshima		
		mild	mod.	severe	mild	mod.	severe	mild	mod.	severe	mild	mod.	severe
-39	M	-	1	1	1	-	-	2	1	2	5	1	-
	F	1	1	1	3	-	1	-	-	-	-	-	-
40-	M	1	1	3	4	-	1	1	2	2	7	-	2
	F	1	1	1	5	-	-	-	-	-	-	-	-
50-	M	1	5	3	3	2	5	2	4	7	6	2	2
	F	1	1	1	1	1	1	-	-	1	1	-	-
60-	M	2	4	10	5	2	9	2	4	10	5	2	-
	F	3	2	2	-	1	1	2	1	2	2	-	1
70-	M	-	2	3	1	3	5	1	-	3	3	-	-
	F	-	2	3	-	2	2	1	-	-	-	1	-
TTL	M	4	13	20	14	7	20	8	11	24	27	5	4
	F	6	7	8	9	4	4	3	1	3	3	1	1
M+F		58			58			50			41		

References

Mukada, T., Sato, E. and Sasano, N. (1976). Comparative studies on dysplasia of esophageal epithelium in four prefectures of Japan (Miyagi, Nara, Wakayama and Aomori) with reference to risk of carcinoma. Tohoku J. exp. Med. 119, 51-63.
Mukada, T., Sasano, N. and Sato, E. (1978). Evaluation of esophageal dysplasia by cytofluorometric analysis. Cancer. 41, 1339-1404.
Sato, E. (1974). Adenomatous polyps of large intestine in autopsy and surgical material. GANN. 65, 295-306
Sato, E., Ouchi, A., Sasano, N. and Ishidate, T. (1976). Polyps and diverticulosis of large bowel in autopsy population of Akita prefecture, compared with Miyagi. Cancer. 37, 1316-1321.
Sato, E., Tokunaga, M., Sakae, K., Mukada, T. and Sasano, N. (1978). Epithelial dysplasia in cancerous and noncancerous esophagi. Tohoku J. exp. Med. 124, 117-128.
Segi, M. (1974). Cancer mortality for selected sites by prefecture in Japan (1969 -1971). Segi Institute of Cancer Epidemiology, Nagoya, Japan.

Epidemiology of Malignant Melanoma in Mexico

A. Mora*, A. Beltrán*, A. Angeles, E. Fajardo*** and
J. Zinser***

**Instituto National de Cancerología of México, Niños Heroes No. 151, México 7.
D.F. México
**Hospital General, S.S.A. of México
***Universidad de Guadalajara, México*

ABSTRACT

660 cases of malignant melanoma were studied; 315 from Hospital General S.S.A.,
232 from Instituto National de Cancerología and 113 from Universidad de Guadalaja
ra. The most frequent primary site was the foot; 34.07%, 35.77% and 40.6% respectively. The possible role of racial and environmental factors in the etiology and
anatomical location is discussed.

(Malignant Melanoma. Epidemiology)

INTRODUCTION

The carcinogenic effect of solar rays is considered an environmental factor in
the etiology of malignant melanoma. Other factors considered are race and heredity. (Elwood and Lee, 1975) A number of the malignancies develop in a pre-existant
nevus. The anatomical location in different races is believed to be secondary to
racial susceptibility and to degrees of protection by melanic pigment (Mc Govern,
1977; Teppo and co-workers' 1978). For instance the most frequent primary sites
in the Caucasian patient are the trunk, upper limbs and head and neck (Pack and
co-workers', 1952; Teppo and co-workers' 1978; Davis and co-workers, 1966), on
the other hand the most frequent primary site in the non white population is the
foot (Lewis, 1967; Pantoja and co-workers' 1976; Sampat and Sirsat, 1966). The
anatomical location of malignant melanoma related to nevi distribution and solar
ray exposition is studied in a group of Mexican Mestizos.

Brief Historical Data

Historically the Mexican race is comprised of an intermingling of the White and
Black races with the native Indians of Mongol origin. Before the Spanish conquest
the Indian population was approximately 9,120,000. Afterward this number was
reduced to half. The Spanish population doubled and the Mestizo increased
sevenfold. At the present time 85% of the Mexican population is considered Mestizo and the remaining 15% is comprised of Indians. As a result their skin color is
brown (Alba, 1977).

MATERIALS AND METHODS

Central México is located at the 23.27° parallel north of the equator. For this reason it receives a high amount of solar radiation approximately 3900 biological units/yearly (Schulze, 1976).

100 aparently normal Mexican adults were examined for number and location of nevi. Freckles were not included.

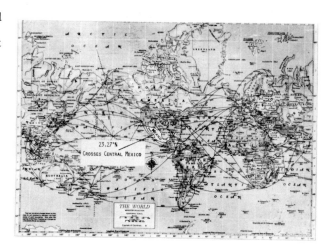

660 Mexican patients with malignant melanoma were studied and divided into three groups:

Group I.   315 cases from hospital General SSA were included. *

Group II.   232 cases from Instituto National de Cancerología were included. *

Group III.   113 cases from Instituto Dermato-lógico and Hospital Civil of Guadalajara were included. *

Fig.1.   23.27°N

Crosses Central México

* Criteria for admission was histological diagnosis of malignant melanoma and primary site location.

RESULTS

Tables 1, 2 and 3 show the anatomical location of the primary tumor in the three groups studied. The skin of the foot is the most common site. Figure 2 shows the five most frequent sites of primary malignant melanoma in Mexicans. They are, in order, foot, upper limb, head and neck, lower limb and oral-nasal mucous membrane. In table 4 the primary site of the disease is compared between the White, Black and Brown races (Davis, Herron and Mc Leod, 1966; Lewis, 1967; Jatin, Shoh and Goldsmith, 1971; Schulze, 1976), The latter includes Puerto Rican, Hindu, and Mexican (Pantoja, Llobert and Roswit, 1976; Sampat and Sirsat, 1966). Table 5 shows the average percentage of nevi location in 100 Mexicans. This data shows no correlation between the site of nevi and the site of the melanoma.

TABLE 1

PRIMARY MALIGNANT MELANOMA. ANATOMIC LOCALIZATION. GROUP I

315 CASES HOSPITAL GENERAL. S.S.A. (10 YEARS)

Foot	92	(34.07 %)
Nostril. antrum and oral mucous membrane ...	27	(9.99 %)
Upper limb	26	(9.62 %)
Face	24	(8.88 %)
Lower limb	23	(8.51 %)
Anus-Recto	16	(5.92 %)
Skin, torax and armpit	15	(5.44 %)
Skin-Non especified place	13	(4.81 %)
Neck skin	11	(4.07 %)
Vulva	6	(2.22 %)
Abdomen	4	(1.48 %)
Perineum	3	(1.11 %)
Back	3	(1.11 %)
Penis	2	(0.74 %)
Hear	2	(0.74 %)
Vagina	1	(0.37 %)
Larynx	1	(0.37 %)
Scalp	1	(0.37 %)
Eye	1	(0.37 %)
Primary melanoma site non informed (44 cases*)		
TOTAL	315	

* Excluded.

TABLE 2

PRIMARY MALIGNANT MELANOMA. ANATOMIC LOCALIZATION. GROUP II
232 CASES. INSTITUTO NACIONAL DE CANCEROLOGIA
(15 YEARS)

REGION	MALE	FEMALE	TOTAL
Foot	38 (35.51%)	45 (36.00%)	83 (35.77%)
Upper Limb	10 (9.34%)	22 (17.6 %)	32 (13.79%)
Face	14 (13.08%)	16 (12.08%)	30 (12.93%)
Lower Limb	10 (9.34%)	14 (11.2 %)	24 (10.34%)
Oral Cavity and Nostril	8 (7.47%)	14 (11.2 %)	22 (9.48%)
Trunk	12 (11.21%)	4 (3.2 %)	16 (6.88%)
Abdomen	4 (3.73%)	2 (2.6 %)	6 (2.58%)
Eye	4 (3.73%)	2 (2.6 %)	6 (2.58%)
Scalp	4 (3.73%)	1 (0.8 %)	5 (2.15%)
Ear	3 (2.80%)	1 (0.8 %)	4 (1.72%)
Vulva	0	4 (3.2 %)	4 (1.72%)
TOTAL	107	125	232

Table 6 shows the amount of solar radiation in biological units received at different parallels. Although there is a high amount of solar radiation in México (3900 units/yearly) the most frequent site of melanoma is not in the areas exposed.

Group II. Sex male 107 patients; female 125 patients. Average, males 56.5 years; female 60.1 years. Occupation, males farmers 36.3%, females, housewives 81.2%.

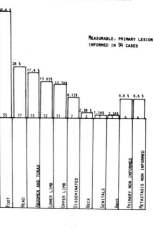

TABLE 3

PRIMARY MALIGNANT MELANOMA. ANATOMIC LOCALIZATION.
GROUP III 113 CASES: INSTITUTO DERMATOLOGICO Y ONCOLOGIA
HOSPITAL CIVIL GUADALAJARA, JAL. (10 YEARS).

MEASURABLE, PRIMARY LESION INFORMED IN 94 CASES

The highest incidence according to age is in the seventh decade. 7101% of all the patients came from México D.F. and the state of México. In this group malignant melanoma comprises 1.26% of all malignancies.

CONCLUSIONS

1. 660 patients with malignant melanoma coming from three different hospitals in México were studied. The foot was found to be the most frequent primary site.

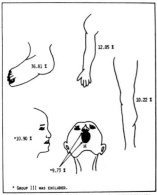

Fig.2. THE FIVE PRINCIPAL ANATOMIC LOCALIZATION SITES OF PRIMARY MALIGNANT MELANOMA IN MEXICAN MESTIZOS (660 CASES) CAN BE OBSERVED IN DIAGRAM.

* GROUP III WAS EXCLUDED.

TABLE 4

MALIGNANT PRIMARY MELANOMA, ANATOMIC LOCALIZATION RACE COMPARISON: WHITE, BLACK,
MEXICAN MESTIZOS, INDIANS AND PUERTO RICANS

LOCALIZATION	WHITE (Queensland)	WHITE (New York)	BLACK (USA)	BLACK (Uganda)	MEXICAN MESTIZOS	INDIANS (Bombay)	PUERTO RICANS
Foot	3.0 %	9.0 % (6.5 %)*	44.0 %	64.0 %	36.81 %	35.29 %	41.17 %
Upper Limb	16.25 %	10.9 %	16.66 %	5.60 %	12.05 %	8.40 %	6.72 %
Face	9.25 %				**10.90 %		
Lower Limb	30.0 %	27.0 %	5.55 %	7.89 %	10.22 %	9.24 %	6.72 %
Nostril and Oral Mucous Membrane				8.0 %	** 9.73 %	15.96 %	
Anus-Rectus					3.54 %	10.92 %	
Back and Trunk	34.0 % (26% espalda)	23.6 %	5.55 %		**4.48 %		7.56 %
Head and Neck	16.75 % (9.25% cara)	22.0 %				8.40 %	29.41 %

* BLACK PATIENTS WERE EXCLUDED
** GROUP III WAS EXCLUDED.

TABLE 5

AVERAGE LOCALIZATION IN PIGMENTED MOLES IN 100 MEXICAN MESTIZOS

	PROMEDIO
UPPER LIMB	2.26
BACK	2.22
FACE	2.13
LOWER LIMB	1.92
NECK SKIN	1.87
TORAX	1.76
ABDOMEN	0.89
FOOT	0.67
HAND AND FINGERS	0.43
EAR	0.36
TOES	0.09
AVERAGE PER CASE	14.6

2. Anatomical site in White, Black and Brown races were compared. The incidence was similar for the different groups in each race. The data suggests that melanine distribution plays a role in the etiology of malignant melanoma.

3. Solar radiation seems to play a lesser role in mexicans (Mestizos) than in the White population.

TABLE 6

GEOGRAPHIC DISTRIBUTION OF ULTRAVIOLET RADIATION (SOLAR AND SKY RADIATION) TOTAL OF BIOLOGIC UNITS PER YEAR

	Monthly Variation Maximum	Monthly Variation Minimum	Biological Units per year
North Pole	9.0	2.5 +1	200
80°N	7.0 +1	1.00+2	370
70°N	8.5 +1	1.24+1	660
60°N	8.4	1.04+2	1100
50°N	8.9 +1	1.18+1	1800
40°N	7.0 +1	1.12+2	2500
30°N	9.0 +1	1.12+2	3200
* 23.45°N	4.9 +2	1.24+2	3900
20°N	4.6 +2	1.57+2	4000
10°N	4.4 +2	2.6 +2	4500
Ecuator	4.7 +2	5.3 +2	4700
10°S	4.6 +2	2.4 +2	4500
20°S	4.9 +2	1.43+2	4000
23.45°S	5.1 +2	1.13+2	3900
30°S	9.9 +1	1.46+2	3300
40°S	9.9 +1	1.53+2	2500
50°S	9.9	1.91+2	1840
60°S	9.3 -1	1.02+2	1140
70°S	9.0	1.29+2	670
80°S	7.8	1.32+2	380
South Pole	9.3	1.68+1	210

* 23:27°N crosses central Mexico. Mexico has a high percentage of Solar Radiation Reception.

Modified from Schulze, R.: Geographic Distribution of Carcinogenic Sun Radiation p. 185, *Cancer of the Skin*. Andrade. Gumport. Popkin. Rees.:Ed. Saunders, 1976.

4. Nevi distribution did not correlate with malignant melanoma in Mexicans.

5. Average age of Mexicans patients is similar to others reported.

REFERENCES

Alba, F. (1977). La Población de México. Evolución y Dilemas (Ed.) Colegio de México, 11-24.

Davis, C.M., J.J. Herron, and G.R. McLeod (1966). Malignant melanoma in Queensland, Lancet 407-410.

Elwood, J.M., and J.A.H. Lee (1975). Recent data on the epidemiology of malignant melanoma. In. J.W. Yabro (Ed.) Seminars in Oncology. Grune Stratton, 11: 2, 149-154.

Jatin, P.S., M.D. Shah, and H.S. Goldsmith (1971). Malignant Melanoma in the North American Negro. Surgery, Gynecology and Obstetrics, 133, 437-439.

Lewis, M.G. (1967). Malignant melanoma in Uganda (the relationship between pigmentation and malignant melanoma on the soles of the feet). British Journal of Cancer, 22, 483-495.

Mc. Govern, V.J. (1977). Aetiology of melanoma. In Milton, G.W. (Ed.) Malignant Melanoma of the Skin and Mucous Membrane. Churchell Levingstone, 1-8.

Pack, T.G., M.D. Gerber, and M.I. Seharnagel (1952). End results in the treatment of malignant melanoma. A report of 1190 cases. Annales of Surgery, 136, 905-911.

Pantoja, E., R.E. Llobert, and B. Roswit (1976). Melanomas of the lower extremity amog native Puerto Ricans. Cancer 38, 1420-1423.

Sampat, M.B., and M.V. Sirsat (1966). Malignant melanoma of the skin and mucous membranes in Indians. Indian Journal of Cancer, 3, 228-254.

Schulze, R. (1976). Geographic Distribution of carcinogenic sun radiation. In Andrade, Gumport, Popkin, Rees (Ed.) Cancer of the skin, Vol. 1. W.B. Saunders Company, 172-188.

Teppo, L., M. Pakkanen, and T. Hakulinen (1978). Sunlight as a risk factor of malignant melanoma of the skin. Cancer 41, 2018-2027.

Melanoma Maligno: Epidemiologia y Grupos de Alto Riesgo

J. M. Iscovich

Fundación Dr. José Maria Mainetti, La Plata, Provincia de Buenos Aires, Argentina

SUMARIO

Las variables intercurrentes en los estudios epidemiológicos de melanoma maligno demuestran la factibilidad de la división en grupos de alto riesgo de acuerdo a 1) asociación/causación estadísticamente asociados y 2) asociación puramente estadística.

El aumento del interés por la génesis de los melanomas malignos fue y es debida en primer lugar a un mayor conocimiento de la evolución de los mismos, como en segundo lugar al aumento, lento pero perceptible, de la incidencia y mortalidad de pacientes con esta lesión tumoral en ciertas áreas.

Los índices de incidencia y mortalidad presentados principalmente en las últimas dos décadas consignan un aumento porcentual por año como simple hecho para poder descubrir esta tendencia, pero hay que recalcar que estas cifras no son válidas para una comparación ajustada ya que los lapsos considerados, la metodología de estudio y el aumento porcentual anual no son constantes.

Sin embargo, es apreciable observar índices anuales que oscilan entre 2,6% y 11,7% para ambos sexos dando una duplicación en la incidencia entre 38 y 9 años respectivamente.

Estas cifras en cierta manera indican que los índices de incidencia aumentaron más rápidamente que los de mortalidad con un rango en estos últimos de 3,7% y 8,2% para ambos sexos, dando una duplicidad de 33 y 14 años respectivamente.

Cabe recalcar, que si la mortalidad de un tumor va en aumento y si este incremento se debe a un factor que en un determinado momento afecta a toda la población por igual, o si aumenta porque mejora el diagnóstico, o porque se deteriora la sobrevida, los índices tienen que aumentar de la misma manera, en todas las edades. Por lo tanto, la curva de distribución de la mortalidad no tiene que cambiar de forma cuando se la compara con edades. Sin embargo, en el caso del

melanoma maligno los aumentos de la incidencia y de la mortalidad fue
ron mucho mayores, en general, en personas jóvenes que en los mayores
de 65 años. Por consiguiente, la edad media de los pacientes que mue-
ren de melanoma maligno está descendiendo.

La diagramación de la mortalidad en función de la edad produce
líneas rectas en escala logarítmica, además la inclinación media de
estas líneas está dentro de la misma gama que la inclinación de otros
tumores estimados sobre la base de datos de incidencia en estudios
transversales, siendo la inclinación para los melanomas malignos la
más baja de todas las registradas. Este índice bajo de incremento no
se altera con lo dicho anteriormente, ya que la escasa inclinación se
debe a un mayor riesgo que tiene la gente joven a través de su vida.

La distribución por sexo de la incidencia de melanoma maligno
varía levemente entre la unidad, siendo más frecuente en el sexo masculino en áreas de baja incidencia, lo contrario sucede en las zonas
de alta incidencia donde la variación es mínima.

Esta diferencia en la razón de sexos de melanoma maligno entre
varias áreas es interesante, ya que otras variables podrían influir
en el hecho de que la razón en el sexo masculino sea diferente. Pero
la diferencia entre sexos estaría enlazada también con la localización topográfica de los melanomas.

En primer lugar es importante recalcar que el incremento en la
incidencia fue mayor en determinados sitios del cuerpo. La incidencia de dichos tumores en la cabeza y cuello aumentó poco en comparación con lo observado en las extremidades inferiores (pierna) de las
mujeres, en el tronco de los varones y en las extremidades superiores
en ambos sexos.

En los datos basados en la incidencia de melanoma maligno en comparación con la cantidad de casos que cabría esperar si la distribución
fuera proporcional a la superficie de la piel, es notorio observar
que las áreas que exhiben excesos significativos de melanomas malignos son en general áreas expuestas: cara, pierna, cuello y brazo en
el sexo femenino; y cara, oreja, cuello y espalda en el sexo masculino. Las áreas que exhiben déficit considerable no están expuestas.
Sin embargo, la frecuencia en el antebrazo y mano masculina es mayor
significativamente a lo esperado. Otros parámetros podrían ser enume-
rados como la frecuencia de melanocitos que varían según la región,
lo mismo que el espesor de la piel; pero los análisis parecen demos-
trar la evidencia que la frecuencia de los melanomas malignos es mayor en las áreas expuestas.

El aumento de la incidencia en las extremidades inferiores de
las mujeres reviste particular interés, ya que la gran mayoría de
melanomas malignos son confirmados en esta localización por diferentes estudios realizados en distintas áreas, siendo su mayor frecuencia en mujeres dentro del grupo etario de 15 a 44 años de edad.

No solamente la localización estaría subordinada a una sola variable dicotómica, esto es exposición o no exposición. Es interesante destacar las diferencias de sitios o localizaciones de acuerdo a
las latitudes.

Los exámenes realizados en **distintos** países o áreas de

diferentes latitudes sugieren que el incremento más grande a medida
que disminuye la latitud se registra en la espalda masculina y en la
pierna de la mujer, o sea en los mismos sitios que exhiben los más
grandes cambios seculares.

Existen no razonables dudas que cuando las sociedades industria
les se desarrollan, la exposición de la población a la radiación solar es mayor. Por otro lado, cabe considerar que los melanomas malig
nos tienen predilección por sitios expuestos, pero esto no es tan de
finitivo como que pudieran derivar de otras partes de la piel y ex-
trapiel. Una simple hipótesis de esto podría ser que los melanomas
malignos tienen dos orígenes: uno independiente de la luz solar y
que aparecería donde existieran melanocitos y otro dado por la exposición. Por lo tanto, el mecanismo por el cual se producen los melanomas malignos por la radiación solar tiene la característica de un
efecto selectivo local y otro general. Las variaciones en la exposición cambian la incidencia, pero alteran muy poco el tipo morfológico
o la distribución del tumor siendo el efecto rápido y no acumulativo.
Por lo tanto, la exposición continuada es compleja y específica en
su relación con los melanomas malignos.

Se ha sugerido que los agentes sistémicos están involucrados,
elaborando la idea del factor solar circundante, basándose en la hipótesis de la existencia de carcinógenos secundarios a distancia de
la piel irradiada.

El otro mecanismo, como posible alternativa, es que el sitio a-
natómico y el tipo patológico de melanoma maligno esté pre-determina
do antes del cambio final hacia la malignidad, basándose en la evolu
ción de clonas malignas de melanocitos anormales. Las radiaciones so
lares actuarían, por lo tanto, como determinante y no como pre-deter
minante de la malignidad.

La clasificacion de los melanomas malignos trae aparejada carac
terísticas importantes. Los melanomas malignos metastisantes superfi
ciales parecerían estar menos asociados a la exposición solar y la
edad media de mayor incidencia es la juventud. Diferente es el lénti
go maligno que es más frecuente en la edad adulta y madurez. Por último, la variedad de melanoma maligno nodular que es invasivo desde
su comienzo, parecería no estar asociada en la topografía a la exposición solar.

Cabe consignar también, que en estudios teóricos y experimenta-
les sobre radiaciones ultravioletas, el ozono juega un papel de fil-
tro de las mismas. Por otro lado, la reducción del ozono por agentes
físicos y químicos como es el caso del cloro-fluorometano podría re-
ducirlo hasta en un 10% en la atmósfera, dando un incremento de las
radiaciones ultravioletas de 19% en latitud 50° hasta 22% alrededor
del ecuador. La relación teórica traería un incremento no solamente
de la incidencia de melanoma maligno sino también de otros tipos de
cáncer de piel. Las mismas consideraciones teóricas darían una curva dosis-respuesta del tipo exponencial.

En un principio vemos que el factor ambiental y el étnico jue-
gan un papel importante en la génesis de los melanomas malignos, por
otro lado, se ha informado a cerca de cánceres familiares con

insistente prevalencia de neoplasias malignas a menudo múltiples o
simples. La tendencia de los primarios múltiples melanomas malignos
entre miembros de familias afectadas y la tendencia de que estas le-
siones malignas aparezcan a más temprana edad, da la sensación de
una labilidad familiar.

Estadísticamente alrededor de 3% de la ocurrencia parece tener
influencia familiar. Son importantes de recalcar dos consideraciones
en los melanomas malignos familiares. En primer lugar la localización, en particular la casi ausencia de localizaciones faciales; y
en segundo lugar la mayor preponderancia de estos casos familiares
en individuos de origen céltico y del norte de Europa. También han
sido estudiados factores hereditarios en relación de melanomas malignos en varias especies animales: Hamster, cerdo y peces.

Se sabe del riesgo de un segundo primario melanoma maligno que
alcanza a un índice de 200 a 900 veces, siendo estos índices depen-
dientes de la edad y el sexo. El riesgo es mayor en la edad juvenil
y en el sexo masculino, en este último casi hasta tres veces.

También ha llamado la atención la co-existencia familiar de o-
tros tipos de neoplasias, habiendo una relación mayor entre melanoma
maligno y cánceres de mama, tracto-gastrointestinal y tumores linfo-
rreticulares.

Otro interesante capítulo corresponde a los melanomas malignos
extra-piel, siendo aproximadamente 1/6 del índice de los melanomas
de piel. Dentro de esta variedad los melanomas oculares representan
alrededor del 35 al 90% de los m lanomas malignos extra-piel siendo
hasta 6 veces más frecuentes en los caucasianos que en los no caucasianos.

El riesgo de melanoma maligno ocular no varía por sexo en compa
ración con los no oculares. Las características geográficas son disi
milares entre los oculares y los no oculares. Se ha visto que los me
lanomas malignos de piel decrecen con el aumento de latitud, parecería que no similar característica ocurre con los oculares.

Dentro de los melanomas malignos oculares hay que hacer una división entre los intra-oculares y los peri-oculares (conjuntivales).
Los melanomas malignos uviales son más comunes en los caucasianos,
siendo raros en los no caucasianos, representando un riesgo de alrededor de 20 veces entre ambos grupos. En cambio, las localizaciones
peri-oculares parecerían ser más frecuentes en las otras razas.

Cabe agregar que en las razas no caucasianas los melanomas malignos de piel representan alrededor de un 35% del total de melanomas malignos en contraste con el casi 80% en los caucasianos, siendo las localizaciones más frecuentes en los no caucasianos boca,
ocular, gastro-intestinal.

Varios estudios demuestran también una agregación familiar en
los melanomas malignos uviales en concordancia con los de piel. El
riesgo se incrementa con la edad y es más alto en la edad madura
aunque existen casos publicados en niños, siendo en general menos
del 4% por debajo de los 30 años de edad.

Por último, la mejor identificación de poblaciones a riesgo de
contraer neoplasias podría estar mejor evaluada cuando la incidencia

es más alta que la correspondiente a los melanomas malignos.

De acuerdo a lo expuesto hasta aquí es posible clasificar los grupos de alto riesgo en: aquel grupo en el cual la variable determinate o pre-determinante tiene una fuerte asociación estadística como el grupo caucasiano dentro del cual el subgrupo céltico tiene mayor riesgo que los demás grupos étnicos; los que habitan en zonas expuestas a mayor radiación ultravioleta, principalmente **dentro** del rango de 295 a 325 nm de longitud de onda; los que tienen familiares cercanos afectados por melanoma maligno, siendo mayor el riesgo cuanto más cercano es el lazo hereditario; también es importante recalcar que los mismos pacientes con melanomas malignos tienen el mayor riesgo de contraer otros malanomas. Y segundo, el grupo con valor estadístico solamente (Figura 1).

Figura 1

VARIABLES DE RIESGO SEGUN ASOCIACION ESTADISTICA

1. Variables asociadas con fuerte valor estadístico

    Caucasianos
    Radiación solar
    Melanoma maligno primario previo
    Antecedentes de melanoma maligno familiar

2. Variables asociadas con valor estadístico

    Ozono
    Otros cánceres primarios (mama, colon)
    Hormonales

Quedando la salvedad que esta clasificación es una aproximación y que su rectificación o ratificación podría modificarse en futuros estudios, en los cuales es menester profundizar en las características del paciente principalmente en el campo de la ocupación y hábitos, en la anatomopatología de la lesión y la exacta ubicación de los melanomas malignos.

Preliminary Investigation of the Epidemiology of Nasopharyngeal Carcinoma (NPC) in Four Provinces and One Autonomous Region in South China

Cooperative NPC Research Group of The People's Republic of China

ABSTRACT

During the years 1970-1975, an intensive retrospective review of death due to NPC was carried out in South China with a population of 170 million. Boat dwellers and migrative population were also included. A cancer registry has been established in Chungshan County to study the variations of incidence and mortality of NPC. Two types of serological surveys (case/control studies and population based surveys) have been carried out to unravel the relationship between the EBV and NPC.

Our investigations showed that the central part of Kwangtung Province including Shaoching, Foshan and Kwangchow districts etc. was a high risk center of NPC with a tendency of decreasing rate toward its periphery. One of the most important features peculiar to the inhabitants living in the above-mentioned NPC high risk areas is that most of them speak Kwangchow dialect. After their emigration to elsewhere, they still maintained a much higher incidence rate of NPC than the local people. In Chungshan County, incidence of lung cancer increased twofold or more during the years 1970-1975, while that of NPC showed no significant changes. Serological surveys pointed to the existence of a parallelism between the presence and development of NPC and EBV antibody titers.

This paper reports our recent research work on epidemiology of NPC in South China.

METHOD OF INVESTIGATION

1. Retrospective survey of mortality rates.

During the years 1970-1975, an intensive retrospective review of death due to NPC was carried out in South China with a population of 170 million covering 453 counties (cities) in Kwangtung, Hunan, Fukien and Kiangsi Provinces and the Kwangsi Chuang Autonomous Region, relying on the concerted efforts of administrative officials, the population and the specialists. 88% of the fatal cases have their diagnosis based on pathological examinations, and the remaining was

81

proved by the typical symptoms and signs with respect to NPC before death. The mortality rates were adjusted according to the age-sex data provided by the national census of 1964.

Two groups of migrative population were also investigated: (1) the nonindigenous people living in Kwangchow City for over 5 years amounted to 109,918 person years during 1970 to 1975, (2) the Kwangtung people having migrated to and lived in Shanghai City for 30-40 years amounted to 182,239 person years during 1965-1975.

2. A cancer registry has been established in Chungshan County since 1970 to study the variations of incidence and mortality of NPC.

3. Sero-epidemiological investigation was done, with 2,300 samples of serum collected and tested by the micro-complement fixation method with antigens prepared from a lymphoblastoid cell line CNL-8.

4. 746 samples of serum were collected and tested for EBV specific IgG antibody to the early antigen (EA) and IgA antibody to the viral capsid antigen (VCA) by indirect immunofluorescence test. The Raji cells and B95-8 cells were used as target cells.

RESULTS

1. The geographical distribution of NPC.

The average mortality rate for 3 consecutive years was 6.53/100,000 population for Kwangtung; 4.66 for Kwangsi; 3.24 for Hunan; 2.66 for Fukien and 1.89 for Kiangsi. The average mortality rate was 4.35 (Table 1).

TABLE 1   Age-sex adjusted mortality rate for NPC
(per 100,000 population) in South China

Province or autonomous region	Age-sex adjusted mortality rate (3 years' average)		
	Male	Female	M + F
Kwangtung	9.05	4.05	6.53
Kwangsi	5.94	2.69	4.66
Hunan	4.37	2.32	3.24
Fukien	4.08	2.17	2.66
Kiangsi	3.07	1.54	1.89

Shaoching (10.4), Foshan (9.71) and Kwangchow (8.98) of Kwangtung Province were the three highest risk districts (Table 2).

Referring to the counties, the highest mortality rate in their respective provinces were Szehui (15.85) in Kwangtung, Pinchiang City (11.14) in Kwangsi, Shuangpai (8.34) in Hunan, Tungshan (7.00) in Fukien and Tayue (5.90) in Kiangsi Province. The lowest risk counties were Huankiang of Kiangsi and Shaoshan of Hunan, both being 0.37, only 1/42 of that in Szehui County.

TABLE 2 **Age-sex adjusted mortality rate of NPC for 1970-1972 in various districts of Kwangtung Province**

District	Age-sex adjusted mortality rate		
	Male	Female	M + F
Shaoching	15.69	5.84	10.42
Foshan	14.21	5.67	9.71
Kwangchow	12.03	4.82	8.98
Huiyang	10.62	3.82	6.24
Shaokuan	8.94	3.59	6.14
Chanjiang	7.49	3.06	5.37
Hainan	8.01	2.63	5.15
Swatow	6.13	2.59	4.31
Meihsien	5.62	1.69	3.44
Average	9.05	4.05	6.53

23 out of the 453 counties and cities had a NPC mortality rate of >9, among them 21 counties were located in Kwangtung Province. Most of these counties (17) belong to Shaoching, Foshan and Kwangchow districts in the central part of Kwangtung Province, the others are situated in their neighbouring districts such as Hueiyang, represented by Tungkuan County (9.33) and Wuchow district of Kwangsi, represented by Tsangwu County (10.74).

2. NPC distribution in the population.

(1) The mortality rate of NPC ranked third to eighth among all cancer mortalities in various provinces. As regard to districts, it ranked first only in Shaoching.

(2) Sex distribution: the average male to female ratio was 1.88:1-2.29:1.

(3) Age distribution: The incidence gradually increased above 20 years of age, with a definite rise for each age group and reached its highest in 50-60 years of age.

(4) NPC mortality rate for boat dwellers was 22.36, much higher than the average level.

(5) The NPC mortality rate (3.64) for non-indigenous people living in Kwangchow City was much lower than that of the Kwangtung natives (10.90) living in the same area. The NPC mortality rate (7.10) of Kwangtung people living in Shanghai was found to be markedly higher than that of the local inhabitants (2.7).

3. Variation of incidence and mortality rates of NPC in Chungshan County (Table 3).

During the period of 1970-1975, the incidence fluctuated between 19.98 and 14.95, averaging 14.68 (20.37 for male and 8.66 for female, with a ratio of 2.38:1), and that of the mortality between 10.31 and 14.32, averaging 12.46 (17.48 for male and 7.44 for female, with a ratio of 2.34:1). The mortality rate of lung cancer during the same period rose from 3.70 in 1970 to 8.30 in 1975.

TABLE 3 NPC incidence and mortality rates in Chungshan County
of Kwangtung Province

Year	Incidence			Mortality		
	Male	Female	M + F	Male	Female	M + F
1970	19.86	8.69	14.24	13.54	7.13	10.31
1971	26.72	9.40	18.02	16.56	8.31	12.41
1972	20.61	8.96	14.74	18.22	7.27	12.69
1973	17.52	8.91	13.20	17.74	6.58	12.13
1974	22.40	7.55	14.95	18.81	6.71	12.73
1975	22.40	8.49	12.98	19.97	8.70	14.32
Average	20.73	8.66	14.68	17.48	7.44	12.46

4. Results of investigations on EBV sero-epidemiology.

90.4% was EBV complement fixation test positive (titre 1:10), with
no significant difference among the various groups of population,
ranging from 87-94%; 12.3% showed high titre antibody (1:320). The
positive rate of 3-5 years age group was 90-100%, with GMT reaching
the peak in various areas. Thereafter, the antibody titre decreased
with age, remained relatively constant during the life span of 20-49
years old, and increased slightly from 50-59. There were no obvious
differences in the level of antibody titres between normal population over 20 years of age in the high risk area (Kwangchow and Chungshan groups), or those in the lower risk areas (Peking, Wuhua and
Lufeng groups), while compared with the high and low risk areas,
significant differences were noted.

5. EBV specific IgG and IgA serum antibodies in NPC.

96% of the untreated NPC patients had IgG antibody to EA with a GMT
of 1:22.7, whereas 5.1% of patients with malignant tumors other than
NPC and 0.9% of normal subjects had these antibodies to EA with a GMT
of 1:1.25-1:1.46. The level of VCA-IgA antibody declined gradually
with an increase in survival time after radiotherapy. Only 30% of
NPC patients had this antibody at very low titers (GMT 1:2.8) 4-18
years after treatment. When recurrence or distant metastasis occured, this antibody increased again and reached its original level.
Consequently it strongly suggested that the EBV was closely associated with NPC.

DISCUSSION

Our investigations showed that the central part of Kwangtung Province including Shaoching, Foshan and Kwangchow districts etc. was a
high risk center of NPC with a tendency of decreasing rate toward
its periphery. Food-stuff, water, rock and soil samples collected
from various areas had been analysed with no definite relationships
found.

One of the most important features peculiar to the inhabitants living
in the afore-mentioned NPC high risk areas is that most of them speak
Kwangchow dialect. After their emigration to elsewhere, they still
maintained a much higher incidence rate of NPC than the local people,
boat dwellers, the earliest settlers in South China, also speak
Kwangchow dialect. They are distributed over the delta of the Pearl
River (i.e. Kwangchow and Foshan districts). Through a long historical period, the boat dwellers had intermarriage with Han people
and most of them are now living ashore. An investigation made recently showed that there remained a rather high mortality rate of NPC.

The inhabitants speaking Southern Fukien dialect in Swatow District
and those speaking Hakka dialect in Meihsien District had a comparatively low rate, being 4.31 and 3.44 respectively.

NPC was highly prevalent in certain families. Among these the Ye-
liang family was a most outstanding example. Among the 49 members
of two generations of this family, there were 9 cases of NPC and one
case of breast cancer. A pair of twin brothers in Hunan developed
NPC in two years. They were later proved to be uniovular twins by
analysis of blood grouping, serum proteins and chromosomal examination of the peripheral lymphocytes. Since 16 years of age the brothers lived in different places of the province. Curiously enough
they had ureter stone in the same year.

In Chungshan County, incidence of lung cancer increased twofold or
more during the years 1970-1975, while that of NPC showed no significant changes. The same was true in Yuehsiu District of Kwangchow
City, the NPC mortality rate being 7.31 in 1964-1965 and 7.91 in
1972-1974; in Shanghai, 1.13 in 1963 and 1.54 in 1975, the increase
being minimal. In South China, childhood NPC cases were rare. Among
the 16,536 cases of NPC diagnosed by the Cancer Hospital of Chungshan Medical College in Kwangchow from 1964-1972, only 19 (0.11%)
were children under 14 years of age, whereas in the low risk area —
Liaoning Province of Northeast China, 41 (4.8%) out of 839 cases were
under 14.

Sero-epidemiological studies pointed to the existence of a parallelism between the presence and development of NPC and EBV antibody
titres.

The results of our investigations suggest that the etiological factors of NPC are multiple, but relatively stable in existence. Hence,
referring to the research work on etiology of NPC in future, a comprehensive study should be made of the chemical, geological and geographical factors as well as virus factors and genetic factors in
particular.

REFERENCE

Lian, C. T. (1974). The geographic distribution and social customs
    of the ancient Yue people. Institute of Genetics, Chinese
    Academy of Science.
Shenyang Medical College (1973). Medical Research (Shenyang), No.
    4-5.
Chen, S. C. (1947). The research on boat dwellers. Commercial
    Press,

Occupational Cancer

Asbestos Cancer in the Construction Industry

A. Englund, G. Engholm and E. Östlund

*The Construction Industry's Organization for Working Environment,
Safety and Health, Stockholm, Sweden*

ABSTRACT

Few studies have been directed towards identification of occupational hazards in such heterogeneous consumer groups as construction workers. Specific trades such as painters, plumbers, pipe-fitters and insulators have definable exposures and an attempt has been made to assess a possible excess of cancer and other causes of death in those groups.

Three cohorts totalling 50.800 have been defined from Union membership records and Certificate records. With the exception 1% of the cases the follow up has covered varying periods between 1965 and 1974 through record linkage with mortality and cancer morbidity registries. The majority of man-years observed occur in young age groups, especially for plumbers and insulators.

The findings indicate an excess of cancer of the respiratory tract in all the occupations studied. This excess is more pronounced in the probably more exposed groups like plumbers and insulators than among the painters. There might be a multiplicative effect of solvent and dust exposure. Oesphageal cancer is found in excess in painters and ventricular cancer in plumbers.

INTRODUCTION

Proper preventive health work requires knowledge about a disease pattern in the group under care. The panorama of causes of death and incidence of different cancers serve as guides to the recognition of hazards to be identified and eliminated.

Few studies have been directed towards identification of occupational hazards in such heterogeneous consumer groups as construction workers. Specific trades like painters, plumbers and pipe-fitters and insulators have exposures possible to define and an attempt has been made to assess a possible excess of cancer and other causes of death in those groups.

MATERIALS AND METHODS

Retrospectively three cohorts were defined. There were 30,580 members of the Painters Union and of employees with certificate for insulation work and plumbing 1,699 and

89

18.521 respectively (Table 1). Such certificates were first issued in 1965 for plumbers and in 1967 for insulators. A person was considered to have entered his cohort when he became a member of the Painters Union or obtained his certificate. Thus the time of entry into the study groups varies among the subjects.

TABLE 1 Size of the Cohorts

Painters	Insulators	Plumbers
30.580	1.699	18.521

The cohorts were followed-up through 1974 with respect to mortality and through 1971 with respect to cancer morbidity. This was possible by record-linking with the yearly death registers kept by the Swedish Central Bureau of Statistics and the Swedish Cancer Registry kept by the National Board of Health.

Such record linking utilizes the ten-digit identification number, which is assigned to every person living in the country. For each person there is a unique identification number.

At the end of the follow-up period each subject belongs to one of the following categories:

- Alive, still living in the country.
  This category could be found in an EDP-file registry kept by the Swedish Central Bureau of Statistics;

- Deceased.
  The category could be found in the yearly mortality registries;

- Emigrated.
  Information about subjects in this category could be found in manual files at the Swedish Tax Authority (Riksskatteverket).

After an initial attempt to assign each subject to one of these three categories, another two groups of subjects with incorrect identifications emerged

- Subjects who erroneously in our file had got identifications of others (false matching);

- Subjects who could not be found in any of the three categories.

Corrections could be made of all incorrect identifications but 50. Thus the loss of follow-up was reduced to 1 o/oo.

Information Available

Through record linking with the mortality files among others the following information items were obtained for deceased subjects:

- Date of death;

- Underlying cause of death;

- Contributory causes of death;

Codes of causes of death are expressed in ICD VII for subjects deceased through 1968 and in ICD VIII for subjects deceased from 1969 on.

From the Cancer Registry the following, among other items, were obtained through record linking.

- Date of diagnosis
- Site of tumour (ICD VII)
- PAD

The original file contained:

- Date of entry into the cohort;
- Cohort-code (painters, insulators, plumbers);
- Date of birth (expressed in the first six digits of the identification number).

The length of follow-up varies among the subjects, the maximum duration extending from 1965 through 1971 with regard to cancer morbidity and through 1974 for mortality. As shown in table 2 the major part of man-years observed falls into young age categories for mortality as well as cancer incidence. The painters have a fair amount of older people in the cohort, while the insulators and plumbers are characteristically young.

TABLE 2   Person-Years of Observation

Age-Group	Mortality Study			Morbidity Study		
	Painters	Insulators	Plumbers	Painters	Insulators	Plumbers
- 19	7928.0	24.0	246.3	6747.9	21.9	235.1
20 - 24	30115.1	856.8	10168.8	20478.1	630.1	7433.1
25 - 29	29213.7	2038.7	19859.1	16929.2	1183.2	12264.9
30 - 34	21602.1	1844.9	19435.3	12564.8	934.6	11962.2
35 - 39	17525.0	1494.6	18312.7	10903.3	826.0	11452.5
40 - 44	14289.5	1333.1	17878.2	9015.1	700.5	11314.3
45 - 49	18047.9	1117.9	16155.3	13415.0	627.2	9828.9
50 - 54	22614.2	889.3	13685.1	15106.0	450.2	8294.8
55 - 59	24322.7	620.9	11900.9	16649.2	348.8	7501.3
60 - 64	21822.5	450.5	9239.1	13494.8	226.5	5378.2
65 - 69	13946.9	195.6	5759.6	7803.9	86.2	3311.7
70 - 74	8169.1	54.7	2503.2	4964.4	10.4	1089.3
75 - 79	4844.9	5.0	462.2	2963.6	3.6	113.5
80 - 84	2268.0	1.6	33.8	1281.6	-	12.7
85 -	776.3	-	6.6	436.8	-	1.3
Total	238025.9	10927.6	145646.2	152753.7	6049.2	90193.8

Each cohort was compared with Swedish males by comparisons between observed and expected numbers of cases. The expected numbers were calculated by using age group (5-year intervals) and calendar year specific numbers of person-years of observation and the corresponding incidence information obtained from official reports concerning Swedish males in reports entitled "Dödsorsaker" (Causes of Death) and "Cancer Incidence in Sweden".

One-tailed p-values were computed using exact Poisson-distributions when the expected number was less than 10, otherwise by approximating the Poisson-distribution with the normal distribution.

RESULTS AND DISCUSSION

Total Mortality and Cancer Morbidity

The total number of deaths in the painter group was 2,740 which did not deviate from the expected number (Table 3). Nor did the 41 deaths in the insulator group deviate significantly from the expected number. The number of deaths in the plumber group, 836, was significantly lower than expected. The total number of cancers in the painter group was 647, which was 9% excess. However, those with more than 25 years between entrance into the Painters´ Union and first year of observation showed a 15% excess in contrast to those with less than 25 years with 2%. Although, the number of cancers in the insulator group was 14 observed versus 9.4 expected, the small number didn´t make this 50% excess significant. Nor did the total number of cancers in the plumber group significantly deviate from expected - 236 versus 211.

TABLE 3 Mortality and Cancer Incidence among Painters, Plumbers and Insulators in the Swedish House Building Trade

	Occupation	Source of inf.	Obs.	Exp.	SMR ·	p-value
	Painters	SCB	2740	2690	1.02	0.18
Total Mortality	Plumbers	SCB	836	939	0.89	0.0005
	Insulators	SCB	48	47	1.02	0.46
	Painters	Cancer reg.	647	590	1.09	0.01
Cancer Incidence	Plumbers	Cancer reg.	236	211	1.12	0.06
	Insulators	Cancer reg.	14	9.4	1.49	0.10

However, the so called healthy worker effect will be marked in a group where selection mechanisms operate and periods of follow-up are short. In addition the plumbers and insulators are observed during a young period of life, when insufficien latency time has been experienced by the people in the cohort.

Although WHO estimated that 80% of the cancers might be caused by environmental factors, only some 5-10% have been estimated to be caused specifically from occupational exposure. There are differences in cancer incidence between urban and rural living areas. Differences in personal habits like smoking and diet also lead to differences in cancer of the lung and of the gastrointestinal tract. There is no reason to believe that Swedish painters, plumbers and insulators differ to an important degree from the typical Swedish male population with regard to factors like urban-rural living or smoking habits. With regard to diet nothing is known.

Specific Cancer Sites

Painters. Among the painters mortality as well as incidence of oesophagel cancer shows a two-fold excess - 24 versus 12 and 17 versus 8 respectively (Table 4). There was a significant excess in deaths from cancer of the respiratory tract with 135 observed versus 106 expected. The same SMR indicating 25-30% excess was shown particularly for the deaths in cancer of the bronchus and the lung. Again the same SMR was shown for the 81 painters reported to the Cancer Registry with cancer of the bronchus and the lung. The excess in cancers of the larynx was higher with 14 observed and 7.9 expected, due to the limited number the significance was not of the same magnitude.

TABLE 4 Gastrointestinal and Respiratory Cancer among Painters

Diagnosis	Source of information	Obs.	Exp.	SMR	p-value
Ca oesophagus (ICD 150)	Cancer registry	17	8	2.15	0.003
Ca oesophagus (ICD 150)	Cause of death	24	12	1.95	0.0005
Ca resp. tract (ICD 160-163)	Cause of death	135	106	1.28	0.003
Ca pulm (ICD 162)	Cancer registry	81	63	1.28	0.01
Ca pulm (ICD 162)	Cause of death	124	98	1.27	0.005
Ca larynx (ICD 161)	Cancer registry	14	8	1.77	0.03

The moderate excess of cancer in the larynx and the lung among the painters and in deaths from non-malignant respiratory disease like bronchitis, emphysema and asthma might be related to previous occupational exposure but the etiology is not known to us. It has, however, been observed that painters have a rate of positive findings on routine X-ray examinations of the lung in our surveillance programs that are higher than we would expect when comparing with people from occupations with higher dust exposure. The disease pattern among the painters also shows an excess in cancer of the oesophagus, larynx and intrahepatic bile ducts, and in addition an excess in mortality from non-malignant diseases in the upper gastrointestinal tract. This pattern is consistent with the finding of an excess in deaths due to alcoholism, but not consistent with the non-excess of liver cirrhosis in the same occupational group. One possibility that has to be ruled out is, that exposure to solvents has caused a typical alcohol-related disease panorama. To what extent the combined exposure to solvent and dust has a multiplicative effect on the respiratory tract is not known to us.

Insulators and plumbers. Generally, the number of deaths or cases reported to the Cancer Registry in single diagnostic areas are low in the insulator group. In spite of that, the number of deaths from tumours in the respiratory tract was 6 versus 1.9 expected, which means slightly more than three-fold excess (Table 5).

In the plumber and pipe-fitter group there was an almost two-fold excess in deaths from tumours of the respiratory tract-81 observed and 41 expected . The same magnitude

of excess, which is highly significant, is shown in particular for deaths form cancer
of the bronchus and lung. 72 observed and 38 expected (Table 5). During the more
limited period of observation a lower number of cases has been reported to the
Cancer Registry - 38 reported versus 24 expected. However, 8 cases of cancer of the
larynx has been reported versus 3.3 expected, which means more than a two-fold
excess in this cancer site. There is a 25% excess in deaths from cancer of the
gastrointestinal tract among the plumbers - 97 observed and 78 expected. In deaths
due to cancer of the ventriculum in particular this excess is 40% - 35 observed
and 25 expected. The excess is more prominent with regard to cancers of the ventriculum reported to the Cancer Registry - 30 reported versus 17 expected.

TABLE 5 Gastrointestinal and Respiratory Cancer: Plumbers, Insulators

Diagnosis	Occupation	Source of inf.	Obs.	Exp.	SMR	p-value
Ca ventr. (ICD 151)	Plumbers	Cancer reg.	30	17	1.72	0.001
Ca ventr. (ICD 151)	Plumbers	Cause of death	35	25	1.39	0.03
Ca larynx (ICD 161)	Plumbers	Cancer reg.	8	3	2.46	0.02
Ca pulm (ICD 162)	Plumbers	Cancer reg.	38	24	1.61	0.002
Ca pulm (ICD 162)	Plumbers	Cause of death	72	38	1.89	<0.0001
Ca resp. tract (ICD 160-163)	Insulators	Cause of death	6	1.9	3.20	0.01

There are some cancer sites where the number of observed cases are small but where
the magnitude of the SMR is high. Such cases are 5 nasal sinus tumours among plumbers and insulators reported to the Cancer Registry to be compared with 1 expected.
Similarly, the number of pancreas tumours reported to the Cancer Registry among
insulators was 4 to be compared with 0.3 expected. The number of deaths from tumours
of the peritoneum (ICD 158) among the painters was 5 against 1.4 expected (p =
0.02) for those who joined the Union more than 25 years ago.

The finding of an excess in respiratory tract cancer amoung plumbers and insulators
is less suprising. The excess is found from the very beginning in the nasal
sinus through the larynx down to the lungs and the pleura. One reasonable explanation could be exposure to asbestos in the past as such an exposure has been
shown in previous studies to cause cancer in the lung and mesothelioma of the
pleura in similar occupational groups by Selikoff (1964). Also among cancers of
the larynx Newhouse (1973) found a relation to exposure to asbestos. So far no
one has reported an excess of nasal sinus tumours due to asbestos or other fiber
exposures. - To what extent the excess in gastrointestinal cancer and above all
ventricular cancer has a similar etiology is not clear to us. However, a similar
finding has been reported previously by Selikoff (1973), among insulators and
also in other studies of asbestos exposure groups.

The data so far reported show findings in a purely statistical analysis. We are at
present examining in detail information from hospital records with regard to parti-
culars of the diagnosis and trying to estimate previous exposures is an attempt to
identify the products and substances that caused the disease at hand.

REFERENCES

Newhouse, M.L., G. Berry (1973). Asbestos and laryngeal carcinoma. Lancet, 2, 615.

Selikoff, I.J., E.C. Hammond (1964). Asbestos exposure and neoplasia. J. Amer. Med. Ass, 188, 22.

Selikoff, I.J., E.C. Hammond, H. Seidman (1973). Cancer risk of insulation workers in the United States. In P. Bogovski, J.C. Gibson, V. Timbrell and J.C. Wagoner (Eds.), Biological effects of asbestos, IARC, Lyon.

Current Status of Cancer Risk in the Rubber Industry

J. A. H. Waterhouse

Birmingham Regional Cancer Registry, Queen Elizabeth Medical Centre, Birmingham B15 2TH, U.K.

ABSTRACT

Case and his colleagues, in a series of classical papers, described the epidemiological evidence for the link between bladder cancer and exposure to beta-naphthylamine in the British chemical and rubber industries. In consequence of this work, beta-naphthylamine was banned for use in anti-oxidants for the rubber industry in 1949.

The present paper describes the results of an investigation conducted in the British rubber industry for two principal reasons: first, to discover whether the banning of beta-naphthylamine had eliminated the excess of bladder tumours; and secondly, to discover whether there were other carcinogenic hazards in the industry.

The answer to the first question is affirmative, but it is only possible to demonstrate the fact by use of a sensitive epidemiological technique which makes allowance for latent period in the induction of the disease. The answer to the second question is probably also in the affirmative, but the size of the excess risk is smaller than that for bladder cancer, and the sites are probably lung and stomach. Further investigation is required, to confirm (or refute) this finding, as well as to localise it by type of occupation, and the study is being continued for this reason.

Earlier Work

It is now well over a quarter of a century ago since Case and his co-workers[1,2,3] demonstrated clearly and conclusively the relationship between beta-naphthylamine and bladder cancer among workers exposed to it. Their investigations had been conducted in the British Chemical Industry, and also in the British Rubber Industry, where beta-naphthylamine was a constituent of the most commonly used anti-oxidants at the time. As a result of his work the substance was banned from industrial use from the end of 1949, and, furthermore bladder cancer was recognised as an industrial disease for which compensation was payable to workers who developed it.

Case's studies had been meticulous and thorough - he had gone to great lengths to
trace every worker; to collect the maximum information about the kind of work
involved; and to consider possible alternative hypotheses. In these respects, it
was a model investigation; and in the early days of analytical epidemiology, it
was also a pioneering study, and justly deserves the epithet "classical", which is
often applied to it.

Proof of Carcinogenicity

The ultimate test of any direct aetiological hypothesis, however securely based,
is the demonstration that removal of the postulated causative agent results in
cessation of the linked disease - or at least a return to its rate of sporadic
occurrence in the population at large. In the case of a malignant disease, with a
long latent period, of the order of twenty years, this kind of demonstration has
to await the passage of time. Workers exposed before the ban took effect could go
on to develop the disease at any subsequent time; and by the same token, an appropriate lapse of time - twenty or more years - would have to ensue before it would
become possible to discover whether workers entering the industry *after* the
imposition of the ban, failed to show an excess of bladder cancer.

Present Investigation

An opportunity to conduct just such a follow-up study came to me a few years ago,
when I was invited by the British Rubber Manufacturers' Association (BRMA) to
undertake an epidemiological investigation of the major tyre factories in the
United Kingdom. The objective was to examine the whole mortality experience of
the industry in the postwar period, rather than being limited to malignant disease.
Nonetheless, the chief interest lay in the cancers, partly in order to be able to
show, if possible, that the excess bladder cancer risk had been removed with the
banning of beta-naphthylamine; and partly because two small-scale unpublished
proportionate mortality studies had suggested a possible increase in two other
sites of cancer. Having experienced painfully the costs of compensation for its
bladder cancer risk, the industry was keen to know about any further possible
hazards as soon as possible.

Design of Study

It was decided to divide the employees entering the factories after the war into
three five-year entry cohorts: first, those entering in the period from 1st
January 1946 to 31st December 1950; secondly, those entering between 1st January
1951 and 31st December 1955; and for the third cohort, those entering between
1st January 1956 and 31st December 1960. The study was limited to males only, and
each factory supplied, in collaboration with our own investigators, the identification details we required, including a description, with dates, of their employment
history. The three entry cohorts referred only to men entering the industry *for
the first time* between the dates specified; and only those who remained for a
minimum period of twelve months were included. Every effort was made to ensure
that no individual who met these criteria was omitted.

Having established retrospectively the composition of each of the three entry
cohorts, the study was of the prospective type, and it remained only to establish
the vital status of each man at the closure date of the study, which was chosen
to be 31st December 1970. The individuals of each cohort fell into three classes:
those known to be alive, perhaps because they were still in employment, or were
currently included in a company pension scheme; those known to be dead, and for

whom the causes of death were known; and the third group whose status was unknown.
In tracing this last group, we were able to make use of both the National
Insurance scheme records - concerned with each man's employment, unemployment or
national pension - and the National Health Service Central Register, concerned
primarily with the administration of the general practitioner section of the Health
Service. We were also furnished, by the Registrar General, with a copy of the
death certificate, in cases where we knew the date, but not the causes, of death.
By extreme diligence, not only on our own part, but on the part of both national
registers, it was possible to trace 98.6% of all the men in the study population.
Table 1 shows the size of each cohort, and its status at the closure date, and
Table 2 shows the efficiency of tracing for each cohort.

TABLE 1   Composition of Entry Cohorts by Status at Closure Date (31.12.70)

	Cohort 1	Cohort 2	Cohort 3	All Cohorts	%
Left & Retired	11007	7120	5421	23548	(63.3)
Currently Employed	3216	2822	3264	9302	(25.0)
Deceased	2660	1182	529	4371	(11.7)
Total	16883	11124	9214	37221	(100.0)

TABLE 2   Efficiency of Tracing for each Entry Cohort

	Cohort 1	Cohort 2	Cohort 3	All Cohorts
No. untraced	292	166	66	524
% Traced	(98.3)	(98.5)	(99.3)	(98.6)

Occupational groups.   An earlier study on Health in the Rubber Industry[4] - a study
of sickness absence records, in which I had also taken part - had defined ten
major occupational groups in the industry, numbered from 1 to 10. In the tabulations which follow, a man whose employment history included work for a minimum of
twelve months in each of two or more of these groups would contribute experience
to more than one group: for this reason the sum of the deaths across occupational
groups will not always correspond with the total for all occupational groups.

Computation of expectations.   From the data available to us, on the date of entry
and birthdate of each employee, we were able to compute, by use of the published
data from the Registrar General, expected figures for the numbers of deaths by
cause, cohort, occupational group, etc., for comparison with the numbers of deaths
observed. The actual comparison is expressed as an "SMR" - a Standardised
Mortality Ratio - in which the observed number of deaths within any subgroup
appears as a percentage of the expected number. An SMR of 100 thus shows complete
agreement between observed and expected numbers of deaths. The statistical significance of differences between observed and expected numbers has been assessed,
using in general the Poisson test. In the tabulations, one, two, or three
asterisks have been set against differences which are statistically significant at
the 5%, 1%, or 0.1% levels, respectively in accordance with contemporary custom.

J. A. H. Waterhouse

"Urban correction" It is well known that mortality in large industrial conurbations is often higher than the national average - and indeed that variations by cause may exist in relation to the size and situation of urban communities. It is possible to use mortality experience for a number of such subdivisions from the publications of the Registrar General for England and Wales, and we therefore used the appropriate rates to correspond individually to each of our participating factories. A footnote appears in those tables where it was possible to make this adjustment.

TABLE 3 Mortality by Occupational Group - All Causes†

		1	2	3	4	5	6	7	8	9	10	ALL
I	O/E	63/61.3	274/285.1	93/126.6	297/305.5	809/1011.9	302/358.8	101/115.5	179/219.4	307/346.2	533/609.3	2571/2924.6
	SMR	102.8	96.1	73.5**	97.2	80.0***	84.2**	87.4	81.6**	88.7*	87.5**	87.9***
II	O/E	18/18.2	120/114.3	51/63.9	87/111.3	365/449.5	149/177.2	51/59.2	87/102.9	151/171.9	195/217.3	1111/1273.4
	SMR	98.7	105.0	79.8	78.2*	81.2***	84.1*	86.2	84.6	87.8	89.7	87.2***
III	O/E	9/7.2	30/35.1	15/16.2	38/44.8	151/178.4	45/56.5	20/32.8	39/41.2	100/84.7	88/89.2	485/523.2
	SMR	124.9	85.4	92.6	84.8	84.7*	79.6	61.0*	94.6	118.0	98.7	92.7
ALL	O/E	90/86.7	424/434.5	159/206.7	422/461.6	1325/1639.7	496/592.5	172/207.5	305/363.5	558/602.8	816/915.8	4167/4721.2
	SMR	103.8	97.6	76.9***	91.4	80.8***	83.7***	82.9*	83.9**	92.6	89.1***	88.3***

O = Observed number of deaths   SMR = Standardised Mortality Ratio
E = Expected number of deaths   = 100 x O/E

†Urban corrected

Table 3 shows the SMRs for All Causes of death, categorised by entry cohort and occupational group, and it makes use of the urban correction. The most notable feature of this table is to be seen best in the last column: with the single exception of Cohort III, the overall SMRs are all statistically very highly significantly below 100. This is the well-known "Healthy Population Effect", found almost invariably in studies especially of manual workers, where the demands of the employment require a fit and healthy individual. To this extent therefore it is a selected population, excluding the chronic sick or disabled, and thus it is likely to exhibit a better mortality experience than the population at large, with which it is being compared. The size of the effect - about 10% - is similar to that found in other industrial studies.

The next table (Table 4) shows, in similar format, the results for Respiratory Disease - this is of course Chapter VIII of the ICD, and excludes lung cancers. Nothing of general importance emerges from this table, so let us pass on to the next (Table 5) - for Ischaemic Heart Disease. Here, nearly all SMRs are below 100, and particularly so in occupation group 5 (the single largest group numerically) concerned with component building. It suggests of course that the active physical work involved here, as in some of the other groups, helps to protect against ischaemic heart disease. In Table 6, for deaths due to Accidents, the majority of SMRs are very low - as they are also in the subgroup of them for Suicides (Table 7). It is valuable, in studies of this kind which may often result in demonstrating serious health hazards in a particular industry, to be able also to show areas of mortality where its experience is better than the average.

TABLE 4 Mortality by Occupational Group – Respiratory Disease†

		1	2	3	4	5	6	7	8	9	10	ALL
I	O/E	15/8.1	46/34.3	15/16.2	47/35.3	116/120.6	34/40.5	19/14.1	23/29.7	62/55.9	80/79.5	391/372.3
	SMR	186.1*	134.1	92.6	133.2	96.2	84.0	134.6	77.4	111.0	100.6	105.0
II	O/E	5/2.3	16/13.3	11/8.4	11/12.5	51/51.4	18/19.6	10/6.9	16/13.3	27/26.7	22/25.5	169/155.8
	SMR	221.4	120.0	130.6	88.0	99.2	91.9	145.6	120.0	101.1	86.4	108.5
III	O/E	1/0.8	3/3.7	3/1.9	2/4.3	11/18.8	6/5.4	1/3.5	3/5.3	16/12.4	7/9.3	48/59.1
	SMR	–	81.4	157.0	46.8	58.5*	111.6	28.2	56.5	128.9	74.9	81.2
ALL	O/E	21/11.1	65/51.3	29/26.5	60/52.1	178/190.8	58/65.5	30/24.5	42/48.4	105/95.0	109/114.3	608/587.2
	SMR	189.4**	126.7	109.3	115.2	93.3	88.6	122.3	86.9	110.6	95.3	103.5

†Urban corrected

TABLE 5 Mortality by Occupational Group – Ischaemic Heart Disease†

		1	2	3	4	5	6	7	8	9	10	ALL
I	O/E	13/15.2	57/71.8	25/28.9	81/75.1	198/242.4	68/87.6	25/28.7	45/53.7	67/83.0	135/149.5	621/708.9
	SMR	85.8	79.4	86.4	107.8	81.7**	77.7*	87.1	83.7	80.7	90.3	87.6***
II	O/E	8/4.8	31/30.2	8/15.3	25/28.7	93/112.1	46/45.0	18/15.3	23/26.9	32/44.1	48/55.2	278/322.1
	SMR	165.8	102.5	52.3*	87.1	82.9	102.2	117.9	85.7	72.6	87.0	86.3*
III	O/E	1/1.9	5/8.8	4/4.1	13/11.4	34/42.5	7/13.4	5/8.4	8/10.6	23/23.0	30/22.9	122/131.1
	SMR	–	56.6	97.7	113.8	80.0	52.2*	59.8	75.4	100.0	131.2	93.0
ALL	O/E	22/21.9	93/110.8	37/48.3	119/115.2	325/397.0	121/146.0	48/52.4	76/91.2	122/150.1	213/227.6	1021/1162.1
	SMR	100.5	83.9	76.6	103.3	81.9***	82.9*	91.7	83.3	81.3*	93.6	87.9***

†Urban corrected

TABLE 6　Mortality by Occupational Group - Accidents, etc. (inc. Suicide)†

		1	2	3	4	5	6	7	8	9	10	ALL
I	O/E	4/4.7	17/25.8	4/11.3	17/31.7	55/104.2	21/38.2	4/10.7	9/16.3	9/15.6	26/49.6	155/259.9
	SMR	84.8	65.8*	35.3*	53.6**	52.8**	55.0**	37.5*	55.4*	57.8	52.4***	59.6***
II	O/E	1/1.6	8/11.3	2/5.5	3/12.2	27/51.3	9/20.2	2/6.1	4/8.2	5/8.6	13/22.5	68/125.6
	SMR	-	70.9	36.2	24.6**	52.7***	44.5**	32.6	48.9	58.1	57.8*	54.2***
III	O/E	0/0.8	2/4.6	1/1.6	8/6.4	10/25.8	8/8.9	1/3.9	3/3.8	4/4.6	5/10.9	37/62.8
	SMR	-	43.5	-	125.8	38.8***	90.4	25.4	78.2	86.5	45.8*	58.9**
ALL	O/E	5/7.1	27/41.7	7/18.5	28/50.3	92/181.2	38/67.2	7/20.7	16/28.3	18/28.8	44/83.0	260/448.2
	SMR	70.4	64.7*	37.9**	55.7***	50.8***	56.5***	33.8***	56.6**	62.5*	53.0***	58.0***

†Urban corrected

TABLE 7　Mortality by Occupational Group - Suicide†

		1	2	3	4	5	6	7	8	9	10	ALL
I	O/E	0/1.4	5/7.4	4/3.5	6/8.2	19/28.2	4/10.7	2/3.1	1/4.7	2/4.7	2/14.1	40/72.5
	SMR	0.0	67.4	113.6	73.0	67.4*	37.3*	65.5	21.1	43.0	14.2**	55.2***
II	O/E	0/0.5	0/3.2	0/1.7	0/3.3	9/13.9	2/5.7	1/1.7	2/2.4	2/2.5	2/6.2	16/35.0
	SMR	0.0	0.0*	0.0	0.0*	64.7	35.1	-	-	-	32.2	45.7***
III	O/E	0/0.2	1/1.3	0/0.5	1/1.7	2/6.5	2/2.3	0/1.1	1/1.0	0/1.3	1/2.9	7/16.6
	SMR	0.0	-	0.0	-	30.6*	-	0.0	-	0.0	-	42.3**
ALL	O/E	0/2.1	6/11.9	4/5.7	7/13.2	30/48.6	8/18.7	3/5.8	4/8.1	4/8.5	5/23.2	63/124.1
	SMR	0.0	50.4*	70.1	53.1*	61.7**	42.8**	51.4	49.2	47.0	21.6**	50.8***

†Urban corrected

Table 8 shows the SMRs for malignant disease, by selected sites and for All Sites, in each Cohort, but for all occupational groups taken together. Bladder cancer is slightly but not significantly raised in the first two cohorts, and tumours of the brain show a significant deficit. There is a successively rising incidence of Stomach cancer, and a significantly high SMR for lung cancer in Cohort III. These we shall proceed to examine more closely.

Latency analysis. Let us first consider the subject of latency. I have already mentioned the time lag between first exposure to a carcinogenic agent and the development of the specific cancer as of the order of twenty years. In order to sharpen the definition of our analysis, and thus to increase its sensitivity, we

TABLE 8 Mortality by Site of Malignancy

		Bladder	Larynx	Pancreas	Prostate	Brain	Colon	Rectum	Lung†	Stomach†	Leukaemia†	All Malignancies†
I	O/E	21/19.3	8/6.0	21/25.7	14/15.2	13/22.8	35/38.2	31/29.0	342/326.4	101/93.9	16/21.2	717/746.1
	SMR	109.0	133.0	81.8	92.0	57.1*	91.5	106.8	104.8	107.6	75.6	96.1
II	O/E	9/8.3	1/2.5	7/11.4	5/6.1	6/10.5	15/16.3	7/12.4	140/139.5	44/39.2	10/10.1	286/323.3
	SMR	108.5	-	61.6	81.7	57.0	92.0	56.4	100.4	112.3	98.9	88.5*
III	O/E	3/3.2	2/0.9	5/4.6	0/2.1	6/4.5	10/6.6	8/4.8	78/54.9	20/14.7	6/4.9	159/132.2
	SMR	92.9	-	108.0	0.0	132.8	151.9	166.3	142.0**	136.4	123.9	120.3*
ALL	O/E	33/30.8	11/9.4	33/41.7	19/23.4	25/37.8	60/61.1	46/46.2	560/520.7	165/147.7	32/36.1	1162/1201.6
	SMR	107.2	117.1	79.2	81.1	66.1*	98.1	99.5	107.5	111.7	88.6	96.7

† Urban corrected

have allowed for a minimum interval of time to elapse within each occupational group before computing the comparison of observed and expected mortality. Thus, deaths from cancer occurring within five years of employment in a specific occupational group would be ignored in a "five year latency period", and *mutatis mutandis* in a "ten year latency period". The refinement introduced by this technique serves to increase the power of detection of carcinogens, enabling the identification of a hazard where its effect may be relatively small.

Table 9 shows the results of this method of analysis, by cohort and occupational group, for All Cancers. The overall total SMR is almost exactly 100, but Cohort III shows a very significant excess, noticeable also in occupational groups 1 and 5. It was only possible to compute a five-year latency for this Cohort.

TABLE 9 Mortality by Occupational Group - All Cancers†

			1	2	3	4	5	6	7	8	9	10	ALL
I	5	O/E	13/14.3	71/62.7	20/27.7	74/67.8	198/220.6	87/76.8	32/25.6	49/49.5	65/75.7	128/138.3	644/643.9
		SMR	91.2	113.3	72.2	109.1	89.8	113.4	125.0	99.1	85.9	92.5	100.0
	10	O/E	10/10.5	54/47.3	15/21.7	57/51.6	160/166.6	69/57.7	23/19.2	39/38.2	44/56.4	96/103.1	502/486.7
		SMR	94.9	114.3	69.2	110.5	96.0	119.5	119.8	102.2	78.0	93.1	103.1
II	5	O/E	0/3.6	22/22.0	13/12.5	12/21.4	82/88.2	35/34.5	8/11.3	15/20.8	30/35.3	41/43.6	228/251.2
		SMR	0.0*	100.1	103.9	56.0*	93.0	101.3	71.1	72.1	85.0	94.1	90.8
	10	O/E	0/1.9	11/11.9	9/6.9	5/12.8	59/52.0	20/20.0	7/6.4	6/12.1	11/20.2	22/25.2	134/145.6
		SMR	0.0	92.5	130.0	38.9*	113.5	99.8	109.7	49.5*	54.6*	87.4	92.1
III	5	O/E	5/1.2	7/5.4	2/2.5	4/6.3	39/25.6	8/8.2	6/5.2	9/6.3	20/13.2	16/13.1	103/77.2
		SMR	436.4**	131.0	-	63.4	152.6**	97.3	116.5	144.1	151.6*	122.2	133.4**
ALL	5	O/E	18/19.0	100/90.0	35/42.7	90/95.6	319/334.3	130/119.5	46/42.0	73/76.5	115/124.2	185/195.0	975/972.3
		SMR	94.9	111.1	82.0	94.2	95.4	108.8	109.5	95.4	92.6	94.9	100.3
	10	O/E	10/12.5	65/59.2	24/28.6	62/64.4	219/218.6	89/77.8	30/25.6	45/50.3	55/76.5	118/128.3	636/632.2
		SMR	80.2	109.9	84.0	96.3	100.2	114.4	117.3	89.5	71.9*	92.0	100.6

†Urban corrected

TABLE 10　Mortality by Occupational Group – Cancer of Bladder

			1	2	3	4	5	6	7	8	9	10	ALL
I	5	O/E	0/0.4	1/1.4	1/0.6	5/1.5	7/4.7	4/1.6	0/0.6	0/1.2	1/2.2	4/3.2	17/14.9
		SMR	0.0	–	–	331.2*	148.1	246.1	0.0	0.0	–	124.5	114.1
	10	O/E	0/0.2	1/0.9	1/0.4	5/1.0	6/3.1	4/1.0	0/0.4	0/0.9	1/1.5	3/2.1	15/9.9
		SMR	0.0	–	–	503.2**	195.8	390.3*	0.0	0.0	–	142.6	152.0
II	5	O/E	0/0.1	2/0.5	0/0.3	0/0.5	2/1.9	1/0.7	0/0.2	1/0.5	0/1.0	2/1.0	7/5.8
		SMR	0.0	–	0.0	0.0	–	–	0.0	–	0.0	–	120.6
	10	O/E	0/0.0	1/0.2	0/0.1	0/0.3	2/1.0	0/0.4	0/0.1	0/0.3	0/0.6	1/0.5	3/3.1
		SMR	0.0	–	0.0	0.0	–	0.0	0.0	0.0	0.0	–	96.7
III	5	O/E	1/0.0	0/0.1	0/0.1	1/0.1	0/0.5	0/0.2	0/0.1	0/0.2	0/0.4	0/0.3	2/1.8
		SMR	–*	0.0	0.0	–	0.0	0.0	0.0	0.0	0.0	0.0	
ALL	5	O/E	1/0.5	3/2.0	1/1.0	6/2.1	9/7.1	5/2.5	0/0.9	1/1.9	1/3.6	6/4.5	26/22.5
		SMR	–	149.3	–	281.0*	126.0	199.2	0.0	–	27.7	134.5	115.7
	10	O/E	0/0.3	2/1.2	1/0.6	5/1.3	8/4.1	4/1.4	0/0.5	0/1.1	1/2.1	4/2.6	18/13.0
		SMR	0.0	–	–	394.3**	195.7	284.7	0.0	0.0	–	152.7	138.7

Turning now to Bladder Cancer, Table 10 is of particular interest.　Only Cohort I shows any significant excess – the All Cohorts excess in occupational group 4 is clearly due entirely to Cohort I – and though the numbers are small the SMRs are high and statistically significant in groups 4 and 6, and to some lesser extent in 5 – the groups in which the exposure to beta-naphthylamine existed.　Thus the latency analysis clearly demonstrates the existence of the hazard precisely where it was expected, among men first employed before the carcinogen was withdrawn; and it shows also the absence of any continuing hazard after its withdrawal. Notice also the increase of SMR from five-year to ten-year latency, which might well increase further as the natural latent period is approximated.

TABLE 11　Mortality by Occupational Group – Cancer of Stomach†

			1	2	3	4	5	6	7	8	9	10	ALL
I	5	O/E	2/1.7	16/7.3	3/3.2	14/7.7	20/25.1	7/8.7	2/3.0	11/6.0	14/9.7	18/16.3	89/75.5
		SMR	–	219.0**	94.5	182.9*	79.6	80.4	66.2	184.7*	143.9	110.5	117.9
	10	O/E	2/1.2	9/5.0	2/2.2	9/5.3	18/17.2	6/5.9	2/2.1	9/4.2	11/6.7	14/11.1	67/51.9
		SMR	–	179.2	–	170.9	104.7	101.5	–	213.9*	164.8	126.2	129.1*
II	5	O/E	0/0.4	1/2.5	1/1.4	3/2.4	16/9.7	5/3.8	2/1.2	2/2.4	4/4.2	5/4.8	33/28.0
		SMR	0.0	–	–	127.5	165.1*	132.8	–	–	95.6	105.1	117.9
	10	O/E	0/0.2	1/1.2	1/0.7	2/1.3	12/5.1	3/1.9	2/0.6	2/1.3	2/2.2	3/2.4	24/14.5
		SMR	0.0	–	–	–	235.8**	157.1	–	–	–	123.0	165.9*
III	5	O/E	1/0.1	2/0.5	0/0.2	0/0.6	5/2.5	1/0.8	1/0.5	1/0.7	3/1.4	1/1.3	13/7.7
		SMR	–	–	0.0	0.0	200.5	–	–	–	207.9	–	167.9
ALL	5	O/E	3/2.3	19/10.3	4/4.8	17/10.6	41/37.3	13/13.3	5/4.8	14/9.0	21/15.4	24/22.3	135/111.2
		SMR	133.6	184.1**	83.4	160.1*	109.9	98.1	104.9	155.9	136.8	107.4	121.4*
	10	O/E	2/1.4	10/6.2	3/2.9	11/6.5	30/22.3	9/7.8	4/2.7	11/5.5	13/8.9	17/13.5	91/66.4
		SMR	–	161.4	103.0	168.7	134.6	115.1	149.2	201.7*	146.1	125.6	137.1***

†Urban corrected

Table 11 examines Stomach cancer in a similar way, and shows some evidence of a significant increase. Again we find the SMR increasing from the five-year to ten-year latency period, especially in Group 5. Cohort III shows also some high though not statistically significant SMRs, where it would be valuable to see the ten-year latency figures. Table 12 refers to Lung cancer, and again shows high SMRs for Cohort III.

TABLE 12 Mortality by Occupational Group - Cancer of Lung†

		1	2	3	4	5	6	7	8	9	10	ALL
I	5 O/E	7/6.3	33/26.2	10/11.0	33/28.5	96/91.0	38/30.3	23/10.8	22/21.6	28/35.6	63/61.0	308/273.5
	SMR	110.7	126.0	91.3	115.7	105.5	125.3	213.7***	102.0	78.7	103.3	112.6*
	10 O/E	5/4.4	29/17.8	7/7.9	26/19.6	78/62.0	28/20.1	15/7.3	19/15.7	20/26.5	48/42.0	248/190.5
	SMR	114.8	162.7**	88.8	132.4	125.9*	139.5	205.4**	121.1	75.5	114.4	130.2***
II	5 O/E	0/1.5	14/8.9	5/5.0	7/8.4	34/35.2	18/13.5	5/4.5	8/8.9	16/16.6	18/18.0	109/103.4
	SMR	0.0	156.9	99.5	83.1	96.5	133.3	110.3	89.9	96.6	99.8	105.4
	10 O/E	0/0.7	6/4.2	3/2.5	3/4.6	24/18.9	10/6.9	4/2.3	2/4.8	4/9.2	7/9.4	55/54.8
	SMR	0.0	141.9	121.2	65.4	127.3	144.8	175.5	41.5	43.3*	74.3	100.4
III	5 O/E	2/0.5	3/2.0	2/1.0	3/2.3	17/9.4	5/2.9	3/2.1	5/2.6	9/6.1	7/5.0	47/30.1
	SMR	-	149.3	-	132.8	181.1*	173.2	145.8	195.8	147.0	140.0	156.4**
ALL	5 O/E	9/8.2	50/37.1	17/16.9	43/39.2	147/135.6	61/46.7	31/17.4	35/33.0	53/58.3	88/84.1	464/406.9
	SMR	109.3	134.7*	100.3	109.7	108.4	130.6*	178.6**	106.0	91.0	104.7	114.0**
	10 O/E	5/5.1	35/22.1	10/10.4	29/24.2	102/80.8	38/27.0	19/9.6	21/20.5	24/35.7	55/51.4	303/245.3
	SMR	98.6	158.7**	96.5	119.7	126.2*	140.9*	198.3**	102.4	67.2*	107.0	123.5***

†Urban corrected

We have looked at a number of other sites of cancer, but these are the most important for the Rubber industry in Britain. While it is gratifying and important that the Bladder cancer hazard no longer exists, it seems that new hazards may be causing excesses of lung and stomach cancer. We are currently investigating these possibilities by extending the closure date by five years; by adding a fourth entry cohort; and by detailed studies of the factory internal environments.

REFERENCES

1. Case, R.A.M. (1953). Incidence of death from tumours of the urinary bladder. *Brit.J.Prev.Soc.Med.*, 7, 14.

2. Case, R.A.M., and Hosker, M.E. (1954). Tumours of the urinary bladder as an occupational disease in the rubber industry in England and Wales. *Ibid.*, *8*, 39.

3. Case, R.A.M., Hosker, M.E., MacDonald, D.B., and Pearson, J.T. (1954). Tumours of the urinary bladder in workmen engaged in the manufacture and use of certain dye stuff intermediate in the chemical industry. *Brit.J.Industr.Med.*, *11*, 75.

4. Parkes, H.G. (1966) *Health in the Rubber Industry: A pilot study*. Rubber Manufacturing Employers' Association.

Co-carcinogenesis in Occupational Cancer

E. Hecker*, H. J. Opferkuch and W. Adolf

*Institut für Biochemie, Deutsches Krebsforschungszentrum,
Im Neuenheimer Feld 280, 6900 Heidelberg, F.R.G.*

ABSTRACT

Plants of the spurge and mecereon families (Euphorbiaceae and Thymelaeaceae, respectively) are used for many horticultural purposes. Most of these species are known to contain highly active irritants. The possibility of carcinogenic risk involved in utilization of these plants is evaluated by isolation and identification of the chemical nature of the irritants and by determination of their tumor promoting activity in mouse skin. The irritants involved were found to be diterpene esters most of them being cocarcinogens of the tumor promoter type. As a result of present investigations it is concluded that qualitatively an occupational hazard might exist for professional gardeners exposed intensively and chronically to irritant species of the plant families incriminated. It is proposed to evaluate the possibility of carcinogenic risk quantitatively by both retrospective and prospective epidemiological studies of groups at risk.

KEY WORDS

Occupational cancer, cocarcinogens of the tumor promoter type, professional gardeners at risk, epidemiological studies, irritant diterpene esters.

INTRODUCTION

According to the wellknown estimate of the World Health Organisation between 75 and 85% of all cancers of human beings are related to environmental factors (WHO, 1964). For most of these human cancers the specific risk factor(s) involved are unknown. Of all cancers those of occupational etiology comprise 1-5% (WHO, 1977). Indeed, careful investigations of occupational cancers have contributed a great deal to identify environmental carcinogenic risk factors, especially those comprising a first order carcinogenic risk such as certain types of irradiation, polycyclic aromatic hydrocarbons (PAH), aromatic amines, vinylchloride and others. Experimentally these factors or certain of their metabolites are known to exhibit mutagenic and/or alkylating properties. It was proposed to collectively call such risk factors solitary carcinogens (Hecker, 1976).

[+]Dedicated to Prof. Dr. med. G. Wagner on occasion of his 60th birthday.

Since about 1966 based on animal experiments evidence was accumulated to indicate that in addition to the classical first order carcinogenic risk factors in the etiology of human cancer also second order carcinogenic risk factors have to be considered which are collectively called co-carcinogens (Hecker, 1976). Although not carcinogenic by themselves, they modulate the effects of subcarcinogenic doses of solitary carcinogens (initiation) to produce tumors in processes called either initiation modification or initiation promotion (Hecker, 1978).

The most potent cocarcinogens hitherto known are the polyfunctional diterpene esters of the promoter type originating from certain plant species or products of such plants (for recent reviews see Hecker, 1978; Evans and Soper, 1978). As far as investigated as yet, they are derived from three different but chemically related diterpene parent hydrocarbons tigliane, ingenane and daphnane (Fig. 1). Usually, polyfunctional diterpene esters of this type are highly active as irritants, as for

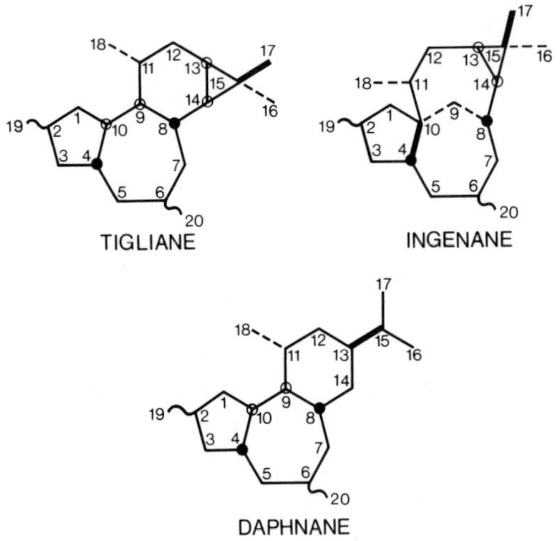

Fig. 1. The diterpene parents of the biologically active principles of Euphorbiaceae and Thymelaeaceae.

example, the croton oil factor A 1. It is a derivative of the diterpene hydrocarbon tigliane, was classified chemically as 12-O-tetradecanoylphorbol-13-acetate (TPA, Fig. 2) and has become the standard promoter in experimental cancer research. Experimentally promoters of this type or their metabolites detected as yet are neither mutagens nor alkylating agents (Hecker, 1978). The polyfunctional diterpene parent of TPA, phorbol, is neither irritant and practically non-promoting in mouse skin (for review see Hecker, 1978). Phorbol was reported to be a promoter of some internal organs of mice and rats if administered after certain solitary carcinogens as initiators (for review see Hecker, 1978). Often but not always, besides the promoters of the TPA type, an additional new kind of cocarcinogen may occur in certain plants or plant products called "cryptic promoters". Thus, for example, in croton oil 50% of its phorbol content is represented as "cryptic promoters" (Hecker, 1978). The typical structure of a cryptic promoter carries an additional ester group in position 20 of the diterpene skeleton (Fig. 2). Upon testing in animal experiments, cryptic promoters do not show impressive irritant or promoting activities. However, by selective enzymatic scission of the ester group in position 20 the corresponding promoters may be cleaved to a highly active promoter. Therefore, as environmental risk factors, cryptic promoters may be even more dangerous than promoters because

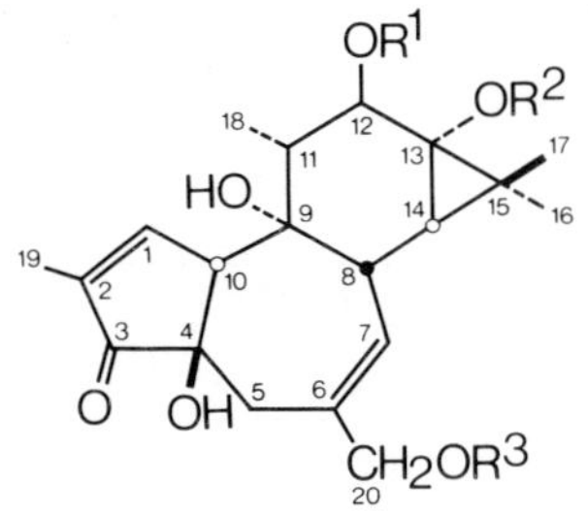

Phorbol: $R^1 = R^2 = R^3 = H$ inactive
Croton Oil Factor A_1 (TPA): $R^1 = CO(CH_2)_{12}CH_3$ promoter
$R^2 = COCH_3$; $R^3 = H$
TPA-20-ester: $R^1 =$ and R^2 as in TPA   cryptic
$R^3 = COR'$ promoter

Fig. 2 The cocarcinogen (promoter) Croton oil factor A1 (TPA),
its diterpenoid parent alcohol phorbol and the corresponding cryptic cocarcinogen (cryptic promoter).

in actual assays their activity is more difficult to detect.

The promoters and cryptic promoters of the diterpene ester type occur in a wide
variety of plant species of the spurge (Euphorbiaceae) and mezereon (Thymelaeaceae)
families, respectively (Hecker, 1968; Evans and Soper, 1978). The source plant of
croton oil is just one species of the spurge family. Recently, evidence was presented that the unusually high rate of esophageal cancer on Curacao most likely is
due to chronic exposure to certain promoters and/or to cryptic promoters of the
tigliane type. Also for this case of human cancer some ideas were developed about
subcarcinogenic exposure to initiators (Hecker and Weber, 1977, Weber and Hecker,
1978).

On the background of these findings and with respect to steadily increasing knowledge as to the occurrence and distribution of highly active promoters and/or cryptic promoters in species of the botanical families involved it appeared worthwhile
to evaluate the carcinogenic risk which may be associated with the utilization of
the species of these families in the human environment, especially in horticulture
(Tables 1 and 2). Many requests to our laboratory from all over the world indicate
that people growing and handling species of the spurge and mecereon families either
as hobbyist's or in a professional manner became alarmed by our findings since
many species of these families are being used as ORNAMENTALS (Table 1), for example,
in family homes, in yards, in gardens and in parks. Many of them are produced in
mass cultures and sold in plant or garden outlets. To mention just a few examples
resentative for the full list of Table 1, the spurge laurel (Daphne mezereum, mecereon family) is a small bush growing in temperate regions all over the world. Early
in spring it flowers beautifully and early in fall it carries nicely red colored
but highly toxic berries of which most of us have been warned by our parents already
as children. The sandbox tree (Hura crepitans, spurge family) is a large tree of
the tropics, especially of West Africa and of tropical South America. Its trunk is
covered densly with thorns and produces an extremely caustic latex and highly toxic
and "explosive" fruits called "sandboxes". In certain States of South America sandbox trees are planted along highways, and several accidents are reported where
people got injured by the poisonous latex which causes severe inflammation upon contact with the skin and temporary blindness upon contact with the eyes. Snow-on-the-

TABLE 1 Species of Euphorbiaceae and Thymelaeaceae used in Horticulture

Scientific Name (Alphabetical)	Family	Common Name in English
ORNAMENTALS		
Aleurites fordii Hemsl.	(E)	Tungoil tree
Daphne mezereum L.	(T)	Spurge laurel
Hura crepitans L.	(E)	Sandbox tree
E.antiquorum L.	(E)	-
E.cyparissias L.	(E)	Cypress spurge
E.ingens E.Mey	(E)	Candelaber tree
E.lactea L.	(E)	Candelaber cactus
E.lathyris L.	(E)	Caper spurge, mole plant
E.marginata Pursh	(E)	Snow-on-the-mountain
E.milii Ch.des Moul.	(E)	Crown-of-thorns
E.myrsinites L.	(E)	Cylinder spurge
E.polychroma Kerner	(E)	-
E.resinifera Berg.	(E)	Euphorbia gum plant
E.tirucalli L.	(E)	Pencil tree
E.triangularis Desf.	(E)	Tree euphorbia
Jatropha curcas L.	(E)	Purge nut
Jatropha gossypifolia L.	(E)	Bellyache bush
Jatropha multifida L.	(E)	Coral plant

mountain (Euphorbia marginata, spurge family), is an annual herb growing preferentially in subtropical climates, for example, in central USA. Its leafes with white margins make them a highly decorative plant for gardens. The pencil tree (E.tirucalli, spurge family), grows in parks and gardens of tropical climates all over the world, showing a remarkable abundance of branches and twigs but only very little if

TABLE 2 Species of Euphorbiaceae used in Horticulture

Scientific name (Alphabetical)	Family	Common Name in English
LIVE FENCES		
E.antiquorum L.	(E)	-
E.milii Ch.des Moul.	(E)	Crown-of-thorns
E.tirucalli L.	(E)	Pencil tree
REPELLANTS		
E.lathyris L.	(E)	Caper spurge, mole plant
FOR SHADE		
Aleurites fordii Hemsl.	(E)	Tungoil tree
Croton tiglium L.	(E)	Purge tree
Hura crepitans L.	(E)	Sandbox tree

any leafes. It is a succulent and therefore becoming popular also as a decorative plant for family homes. - Other species of the spurge family are used for other horticultural purposes (Table 2). Quite a few are used as LIVE FENCES, such as

E.antiquorum, Crown-of-thorns (E.milii) and again the pencil tree (E.tirucalli). The mole plant (E.lathyris) is known to many gardeners as a MOLE REPELLANT. Various other species are planted just FOR SHADE, for example, the purge tree (Croton tiglium), the source of croton oil, to protect coffee plantations from too much of sunshine.

TABLE 3 Species of Euphorbiaceae and Thymelaeaceae of Horticultural Interest arranged according to Diterpene Parent of their irritant Principles

Scientific Name Alphabetical	SPECIES Family	Common Name in English	UTILIZATION in Homes, Yards, gardens or parks
		TIGLIANE	
Aleurites fordii Hemsl.	(E)	Tungoil tree	ornamental, for shade
Croton tiglium L.	(E)	Purge tree	for shade
E.resinifera Berg	(E)	Euphorbia gum plant	ornamental
E.tirucalli L.	(E)	Pencil tree	live fences, ornamental
E.triangularis Desf.	(E)	Tree euphorbia	ornamental
Jatropha curcas L.	(E)	Purge nut	ornamental
Jatropha gossypifolia L.	(E)	Bellyache bush	ornamental
Jatropha multifida L.	(E)	Coral plant	ornamental
		DAPHNANE	
Daphne mezereum	(T)	Spurge laurel	ornamental
E.resinifera Berg	(E)	Euphorbia gum plant	ornamental
Hura crepitans L.	(E)	Sandbox tree	ornamental, for shade
		INGENANE	
E.antiquorum L.	(E)	-	live fences, ornamental
E.cyparissias L.	(E)	Cypress spurge	ornamental
E.ingens E.Mey	(E)	Candelaber tree	ornamental
E.lactea	(E)	Candelaber cactus	live fences, ornamental
E.lathyris L.	(E)	Caper spurge, mole plant	ornamental, mole repellant
E.marginata Pursh.	(E)	Snow-on-the-mountain	ornamental
E.milii Ch.des Moul.	(E)	Crown of-thorns	live fences, ornamental
E.myrsinites L.	(E)	Cylinder spurge	ornamental
E.polychroma Kerner	(E)	-	ornamental
E.resinifera Berg.	(E)	Euphorbia gum plant	ornamental
E.tirucally L.	(E)	Pencil tree	live fences, ornamental

From all species compiled in Tables 1 and 2 irritant principles were isolated containing diterpene moieties derived from the parent hydrocarbons tigliane, daphnane and ingenane and typical for promoters of mouse skin. Thus, for example, the purge and the pencil trees contain tigliane type diterpene esters, while the spurge laurel and the sandbox tree both contain daphnane type diterpene esters (Table 3). While research in this area is still going on, some facts relevant for evaluation of the possible carcinogenic risk involved in growing and maintaining these plants may be summarized:

1. A plant belonging to either one of the spurge or mecereon family must not necessarily contain irritant diterpene esters: Besides the growing list of species of these families with identified irritant principles we do have also a growing list of species which, although belonging to one of these families, do not contain irritant principles ("negative list"). For example, in our "negative list" we carry the wellknown Poinsettia (Euphorbia pulcherrima) in which we did not find any irritant diterpene esters, although samples of this species collected from at least five different localities all over the world were investigated. Therefore, this species seems to be comparatively save for production in mass cultures as so happens, annually before Christmas, in many parts of the world. For at least two other species we found that the content of irritant diterpene esters seemingly depends on some soil and/or climate conditions according to which the plants investigated have been raised: thus, for example, the pencil tree (Euphorbia tirucalli) grown in tropical regions produces one of the most irritant latices known, whereas the latex of the same species grown in the green house behind our institute in Heidelberg, did not show any irritant activity. Apparently, the biochemical machinery producing the irritant diterpene esters (Adolf and Hecker, 1977) does not work in the plant if grown in the soil and/or in the climate of our region.

2. In those plants of the spurge and mecereon families which contain identified irritants - all those compiled in Table 3 - it was found that the diterpene esters responsible for irritancy not necessarily are also promoters of mouse skin. For example, some of the most irritant plants such as E. tirucalli (pencil tree). and E.resinifera (euphorbia gum plant) contain diterpene esters of the tigliane and

TABLE 4 Species of Euphorbiaceae and Thymelaeaceae of Horticultural Interest Irritancy and Promoting Activity of some Diterpene Esters Isolated as compared to Croton oil factor A_1 (TPA) and Pimelea factor P_2

Species	Family	Irritant Factor Name	Type of Diterpene Parent	Irritancy ID_{50} (mmole/ear)[a]	Promoting Activity (rel.potency)[c]
IRRITANTS AND PROMOTERS					
Croton tiglium L. (E)		Croton oil factor A_1 (TPA)	tigliane	$1.6 \cdot 10^{-8}$	++++
Pimelea prostrata Willd. (T)		Pimelea factor P_2	daphnane	$3.0 \cdot 10^{-9}$	+++
IRRITANTS ONLY					
Euphorbia tirucalli L. (E)		Euphorbia factor Ti_8	tigliane	$1.6 \cdot 10^{-8}$	(+)
Euphorbia resinifera Berg (E)		Resiniferatoxin	daphnane	10^{-11} [b]	0

a) irritant dose 50 (ID50) on the mouse ear read 24 h after administration
b) read two hours after administration
c) standard assay for promoters on back skin of mice with DMBA as initiator

daphnane type, respectively (see Table 4), which exhibit irritant doses 50 comparable to or even below the irritant dose 50 of croton oil factor A1 (TPA) or else pimelea factor P2. Therefore, they are comparatively or more active than irritants as TPA or pimelea factor P2, respectively. Yet, these highly irritant compounds do not show any appreciable promoting activity in the standard assay on the back skin of mice.

3. None the less as a rule, the majority of the plants of the spurge and mecereon families investigated up to now contain diterpene esters which are more or less active as irritants or cryptic irritants but also as promoters and/or as cryptic promoters of mouse skin.

On the background of present knowledge, as a preliminary judgement of the carcinogenic risk associated with horticultural utilization of the plants, it appears that the maintenance of single plants of these families does not mean an actual carcinogenic risk if intensive (chronic) contact with the skin or ingestion by mouth is avoided. Measures of this kind are generally valid also for handling of other toxic ornamenals the beauty of which we enjoy although we know that they are toxic. However, the situation appears different with people who by profession are intensively exposed to irritant species of this kind, for example, by handling of mass cultures, by redressing of live fences or by raising crops in the shade of certain poisonous trees. Qualitatively such and similar professional exposure might be considered a potential risk of cancer. To evaluate such risk quantitatively, both retrospective and prospective epidemiologic studies should be started immediately in groups at risk professionally. Investigations of this kind may be especially indicated in view of the fact that besides wellknown chemical initiators possibly also initiators of the viral type may have to be considered: according to a most recent joint investigation of our laboratory together with Prof. zur Hausen and coworkers, from Freiburg, Germany, it was demonstrated that cells containing genomes of the Epstein-Barr-Virus which is not expressed by virus synthesis, may become virus producers to the extent of close to 100 % if they are exposed to promoters of the diterpene ester type (zur Hausen et al., 1978).

REFERENCES

Adolf, W. and Hecker, E. (1977). Diterpenoid irritants and cocarcinogens in Euphorbiaceae and Thymelaeaceae: Structural relationships in view of their biogenesis. Israel J. Chem., 16, 75-83.

Evans, F.J. and Soper, C.J. (1978). The tigliane, daphnane and ingenane diterpenes, their chemistry, distribution and biological activity. Lloydia, 41, 193-233.

Hecker, E. (1976). Definitions and terminology in cancer (tumor) etiology - an analysis aiming at proposals for a current internationally standardized terminology. Internat.J.Cancer, 18, 122-129; see also Z.Krebsforsch., 86, 219-230; GANN, 67, 471-481; Bull.World Health Organ., 54, 1-10.

Hecker, E. and Weber, J. (1977). 7th International Symposium on the biological characterization of human tumors. Budapest, 13-15 April 1977, Proceedings. (1978). Advances in tumor prevention, detection and characterization. In W.Davis (Ed.), Characterization and Treatment of human tumors, Vol. 4, series 420. Excerpta Medica, Amsterdam. pp. 72-75. See also: Weber, J. and Hecker, E. (1978). Cocarcinogens from Croton flavens L. and esophageal cancer in Curacao. Experientia, 34, 679-680.

Hecker, E. (1978). Structure-activity relationships in diterpene esters irritant and cocarcinogenic to mouse skin. In. T.J. Slaga, A. Sivak and R.K. Boutwell (Eds.), Carcinogenesis, Vol.2, Mechanisms of tumor promotion and cocarcinogenesis. Raven Press, New York. pp. 11-48.

WHO (1964). Prevention of cancer: Technical report, Series 276. Geneva, Switzerland.

WHO (1977). IARC: Past and present developments. WHO Chronicle, 31, 239-245, see p. 243.

zur Hausen, H., O'Neill, F.B., Freese, U.K. and Hecker, E. (1978). Persisting oncogenic herpesvirus induced by the tumor promoter TPA. Nature, 272, 373-374.

Setting of Exposure Standards

Bo Holmberg

Unit of Occupational Toxicology, Department of Occupational Health,
National Board of Occupational Safety and Health,
Arbetarskyddsstyrelsen, Fack, S-100 26 Stockholm, Sweden

ABSTRACT

The setting of exposure standards for chemical carcinogens involves many problems of a scientific and trans-scientific nature giving a wide spectrum of levels of action for carcinogens in different countries.

Experimental and epidemiological data indicate that the dose-response curve is linear in the low dose range from zero dose and onwards. Small doses may, however, be more effective per dose unit in producing cancer than high doses. Sometimes an inverted dose-response may also be seen for some cancer types although the dose-response-relationship for all tumors is the classical one.

Animal experiments are performed on "standardized" animals in standardized environment and with one chemical at a time. The human exposure panorama is much more complex and dynamic. Extrapolation from animals to man in quantitative terms is therefore not possible.

The setting of exposure standards means accepting a <u>low risk level</u>. In this decision an evaluation of technological feasibility is also involved. In the absence of a good estimate of the risk level, the technological feasibility may indicate a low exposure level as in the case of vinyl chloride, trichloroethylene and rubber chemicals.

Key words: dose response relationship, mouse-man extrapolations, technological feasibility.

INTRODUCTION

The setting of occupational standards for chemical carcinogens involves many challenging problems of toxicological and trans-scientific (Weinberg, 1972) nature. First of all, we need to discuss the problems of extrapolating dose data from high levels of exposure to low levels of exposure involving questions about the true form of the dose-response-curve. We have also to discuss the possibilities of extrapolating dose data from experimental test systems to human populations. Thirdly, we have to admit that, for most carcinogens, no dose data are at hand for past human exposure and that a decision on the permissible level of occupational exposure, if any exposure level above zero should be permissible, often has to be made in the absence of quantitative dose data. I believe that it is as important to

115

recognize the uncertainties, as well as the certainties, in the difficult but important task of standard setting for chemical carcinogens.

HIGH DOSE TO LOW DOSE EXTRAPOLATIONS

For most toxic substances it is possible to establish a dose which on the individual level does not cause a harmful effect, a so called no effect level. With a decrease in dose the effects will be more and more reduced in intensity and will eventually disappear. For carcinogenic agents no such dose seems to be possible to establish; cancer is an all-or-none-effect. When a transformed cell line is already established, the tumor growth rate is not influenced by increasing the dose of the initiating agent (Saffiotti, 1977). The fact that a no-effect-level cannot be established for the individual is however not contradictory to the fact that small populations can be encountered with no tumors. Such no-response-levels do simply reflect small sample sizes and the biological variability of the population.

Tumor induction tests involve a limited number of animals, say 50 or 100 animals in each dose group. Such a test system cannot detect low-frequent tumors (Zbinden, 1973). In the presence of "spontaneous" tumors in the target organ, the sensitivity is even more reduced (Crump and coworkers, 1976). The low sensitivity of the test system forces the toxicologist to use high dose levels of the test chemical, dose levels which often seem "unrealistic" in terms of human occupational exposure. Thus, extrapolation models are needed in order to predict the carcinogenic risk for the mouse at low dose levels. Such extrapolation models are developed (Schneiderman, Mantel and Brown, 1975) although no one knows which model is the true one. All experimental data obtained with a limited number of animals indicate, however, that a one-hit mechanism (Ehrenberg and Holmberg, 1978) may play a part in the induction of a mutation and of cancer (Crump and coworkers, 1976; Ehrenberg and Holmberg, 1978). This is supported by certain epidemiological data (Report of a Task Group, 1978). Thus, a linear relationship between dose and response in the low dose range seem to fit all data. This means that there does not exist a threshold level for cancer induction or a true safe level of exposure to carcinogens.

The most reasonable assumption is that the dose-response-curves for human carcinogens have the same form as for experimental carcinogens. For asbestos (Peto, 1978) a linear relationship in the low dose area seem to be the most probable. By using Williams' data (1958) on bladder cancer induced by 2-aminonaphtalene and benzidine, the frequency of tumors can be plotted against log dose, or more exactly log time period of exposure (Säfwenberg and Holmberg, 1975). This curve does not significantly deviate from linearity above zero dose. There are too few chemicals available where we have dose response data from both animals and human populations to allow us to make comparisons and to allow us to make meaningful statements on which model is generally valid for all carcinogens, if one single valid model exists at all. For those few chemicals for which a comparison can be made (Cranmer, 1977), a big difference in predicted risk levels is obtained for the same dose of the chemical if human exposure data are used instead of animal dose data. As we do not know which extrapolation model to be used, it has been suggested (Saffiotti, 1978) that the model giving the largest overestimate of risk should be preferred.

When discussing the dose-response relationship it should, however, be mentioned that low doses sometimes may be more effective than higher doses. This has been shown for radiation (Brown, 1976) and urethane (Schmähl, Port and Wahrendorf, 1977). The time of administration of a dose is also known to affect the degree of response to carcinogens. Thus, the fractionation of a dose of a polycyclic hydrocarbon (Payne and Hueper, 1960) or a nitrosamine (Druckrey, 1967) into small subdoses is more effective in producing tumor bearing animals than the same total dose given in one injection. This phenomenon has consequences for the standard setting of occupational exposures as a fractionated exposure is exactly that situation existing in the work environment.

By analysing dose-response data in the litarature one may also find that some tumors are more frequent at low doses than at high doses. Such a paradoxical dose-response relationship is for instance demonstrated for asbestos induced mesotheliomas as for vinyl chloride induced (Table 1) hemangiosarcomas (Holmberg, Kronevi and Winell, 1976). This paradoxical dose-response relationship may be an important pitfall when making risk evaluations based upon epidemiological studies, particularly in case control studies.

Table 1. Dose Response Data of VCM-Induced Tumors in Mice*

Exposure regime	50 ppm, 6 h/d, 5 d/w, during 52 weeks	500 ppm, 6 h/d, 5 d/w, during 26 weeks
"Life dose"	78 000 ppmhours	390 000 ppmhours
Animals with tumors	75 % (18/24)	100 % (24/24)
Animals with more than one tumor	61 % (11/18)	50% (12/24)
Mean number of hemangiosarcomas pro tumorbearing animal surviving more than 6 months	1.7 % (27/16)	0.9 % (14/16)
Tumorbearing animals with hemangiosarcoma, which died spontaneously	88 % (14/16)	50 % (8/16)

*(Holmberg, Kronevi and Winell, 1976)

A reduction of the total dose may also increase the latency period (Jones and Grendon, 1975). This has been mathematically expressed by Druckrey (1967) as $d \cdot t^n$ = constant, where d is the daily dose, t the mean latency time and n a characteristic for each compound and possibly also for each test system. The n-value has been proposed (Jones and Grendon, 1975) to be 3 for most carcinogens. That this is far from true is shown in Table 2, where n-values from some studies are put together. Most of these figures are based upon experimental studies. n-Values for human exposures are obtainable only for a few compounds, such as tobacco smoke (Albert and Altshuler, 1973) and aromatic amines (Säfwenberg and Holmberg, 1975). The n-values from human exposures are among the highest in the entire cancer literature, higher than for any experimental carcinogens. The great variations in n-values suggest that a simple reduction of the dose by 1000 (Jones and Grendon, 1975) for all carcinogens will apparently not lead to cancerfree human populations. It has also been stated (Armenian and Lilienfeld, 1974) that much larger dose changes have to be introduced to significantly reduce the latency period than to reduce the tumor frequency for human response. When considering the extrapolation of dose latency data it is also important to note that the variation in individual latency times is increased by reducing the dose (Druckrey, 1967). This means that even a dose giving a mean latency time above the expectance of life-time may still cause tumors in some susceptible individuals (Ehrenberg and Holmberg, 1978).

Table 2. n-Values for Some Carcinogens According to Druckrey's Formula*

$$d \cdot t^n = k$$

Substance	Tumor/adm.route	n-Value	Reference
3-methylcholantrene	local, skin painting	2.1	Horton and Deman, 1955.
Benzo(a)pyrene	local, skin painting	4.0	Poel, 1956.
Benzo(a)pyrene	local, subcut. inj.	4.7	Bryan and Shimkin, 1943.
Diethylnitrosamine	liver, oral	2.3	Druckrey and co-workers, 1967.
Diisopropylnitros-amine	liver, oral	1.2	Druckrey and co-workers, 1967.
Dimethylamino-stilbene	ear duct, oral	3.0	Druckrey and co-workers, 1967.
Dimethylbenzanthra-cene	local, skin painting	1.4	Albert and Altshuler, 1973.
Cigarette smoke	lung (human) inhalation	8.0	Albert and Altshuler, 1973.
Aromatic amines (benzidine, β-naphtylamine)	urinary bladder (human), inhalation	6.4	Säfwenberg and Holmberg, 1975.

*(Druckrey, 1967)

EXTRAPOLATION FROM MOUSE TO MAN

Human cancer is probably more often multifactorial (Preussmann, 1976; Selikoff, 1975) than caused by one single agent. We are all exposed for initiators and/or promotors from different sources (e g food, drugs, the general and occupational environment). Experimental animals are generally exposed only to one test chemical in their life time and are genetically and environmentally standardized but the human individual is not. The human individual is no tabula rasa. Moreover, many chemicals in our environment might unpredictably influence the response to chemical carcinogens. Extrapolations of dose-response data from one single chemical obtained in an experimental test system to the more complex human exposure situation should therefore not be done in order to establish "safe" levels of human exposure. In the absence of human dose response data, experimental carcinogens should be listed and warned for. The exposure should be reduced to as low levels as possible or the compound be prohibited.

Extrapolation models as obtained on animals with chemicals should be used on epidemiological dose response data. This can, however, in practice seldom be done due to the fact that dose data for past exposures do not exist. So far, good dose data for past exposures exist only for a few chemicals, such as asbestos (Peto, 1978), benzo(a)pyrene (Hammond and coworkers, 1976), arsenic (Ott, Holder and Gordon, 1974), and tobacco smoke (Doll, 1971). In order to get relevant dose data for future epidemiology, we ought, as scientists, to put a demand upon the industry to establish exposure controls for all carcinogens used.

ADDITIONAL BASIS FOR STANDARD SETTING

The discussion leads to the conclusion that dose-response curves for chemical carcinogens probably are linear from dose zero and onwards, which means that safe levels of exposure to carcinogens do not exist. Thus, the setting of an exposure standard for a carcinogen is an administrative decision, which involves the acceptance of a <u>low risk level</u> of exposure (Holmberg and Westlin, 1978). I personally believe that it is important that the workers themselves in some way participate in the process of accepting the risk level as no expert can tell what risk the worker has to accept. The setting of standards in the work environment have for most of the carcinogens to be done without sufficient knowledge about past doses. The standard setting of occupational carcinogens is a typical trans-scientific judgment (Weinberg, 1972), involving also an evaluation of technological feasibility (Holmberg and Westlin, 1978).

The concept of technological feasibility includes evaluations of the strategy for taking air samples, methods of analysis and of hygienic surveillance of the emissions. It also includes evaluations of what is technologically (and economically) possible in an optimal improvement of the work hygiene. It should also be kept in mind that the concept of technological feasibility may not be constant from time to time or from one country to another. What seems not feasible today could well tomorrow be regarded as a minimal requirement. Differences in exposure standards between countries do apparently reflect differences in what is regarded as technologically feasible. Especially in the absence of a good medical risk estimate, but also in its presence, the evaluation of technological feasibility may be decisive in the last run in the standard setting procedure. This was, for instance, the case for trichloroethylene (Hygieniska gränsvärden, 1978), vinyl chloride (Westlin and Holmberg, 1978) and is proposed for certain air pollutants in the rubber industry (Holmberg and Sjöström, 1977). Trichloroethylene is carcinogenic to mice (NCI, 1976) by peroral administration but seems not to represent a high cancer risk for Swedish metal degreasers (Axelson and coworkers, 1978), at least not when compared to vinyl chloride. The normal use of trichloroethylene as a degreasing agent should generally not give exposure levels above 20 ppm (Wettström and Zetterkvist, 1978) as a time weighted average. Thus, the trichloroethylene standard was set at 20 ppm. For vinyl chloride, the production process and the elimination technology, as well as the methods of emission control in the working area (Englund and Holmberg, 1976; Holmberg and Westlin, 1978) could be greatly improved giving a level of 1 ppm as a feasible level.

In the rubber industry around 500 chemicals are used (Holmberg and Sjöström, 1977), such as curing agents, accelerators, fillers, antiozonants, peptizizers, inhibitors and activators. Around 250 of these compounds are either not chemically defined or they completely lack toxicological information or both. Only two or three compounds (mineral oil, trichloroethylene, ethylene thiourea) used in the Swedish rubber industry today are carcinogenic, all of which are regulated by the authority. Around 40 compounds of those used in the rubber industry should preferably be investigated further for possible carcinogenic activity. This is needed because they are structurally similar to known carcinogens, or they are mutagenic in screening tests or may have caused some tumors in conventional cancer tests which are not possible to evaluate definitely. It is meaningless to establish occupational standards only for a few single carcinogens in an industry like the polymer industries and avoid regulating all other chemicals which may still contribute to the overall risk. A more general approach for improvning the work hygiene in such industries is apparently needed. Such may partly be done by turning over from handling of dusty powder chemicals to the handling of pellets, granulates, masterbatch or the like (Holmberg and Sjöström, 1977), or by installing automatic weighing equipments for all chemicals (Olsson, 1977). This will certainly reduce the cancer risk in the weighing and mixing departments of the polymer industry and is an example on a standard setting approach without giving a numerical value for single air pollutants.

REFERENCES

Albert R.E. and Altshuler B. (1973). Considerations relating to the formulation of limits for unavoidable population exposures to environmental carcinogens. In: J.E. Ballow (Ed) Radionuclide carcinogenesis. AEc symp. series conf. - 72050, Springfield, NTIS, 233-253.

Armenian H.K. and Lilienfield A.M. (1974). The distribution of incubation periods of neoplastic deseases. Am. J. Epidem., 99, 92-100.

Axelson O., Andersson K., Hogstedt C., Holmberg B., Molina G., and de Verdier A (1978). A cohort study on trichloroethylene exposure and cancer mortality. J. Occ. Med., 20, 194-196.

Brown J.M. (1976). Linearity vs. non-linearity of dose-response for radiation carcinogenesis. Health Phys., 31, 231-245.

Bryan W.R. and Shimkin M.B. (1943). Quantitative analysis of dose-response data obtained with three carcinogenic hydrocarbons in Strain C3H male mice. J. Nat. Cancer inst. 3, 503-531.

Cranmer M.F. (1977). Estimation of risks due to environmental carcinogenesis. Med. Ped. Oncol., 3, 169-198.

Crump K.S., Hoel D.G., Langley C.H. and Peto R. (1976). Fundamental carcinogenic processes and their implications for low dose risk assessment. Cancer Res., 36, 2973-2979.

Doll R. (1971) Cancer and aging: The epidemiologic evidence. In: Tenth international cancer congress, Houston, May 22-29 1970. Oncology 1970. Year book medical publ. Inc., Chicago, 133-160.

Druckrey H. (1967). Quantitative aspects in chemical carcinogenesis. In: R. Truhaut (Ed.), UICC Monograph series vol. 7. Potential carcinogenic hazards from drugs. Evaluation of risks. Springer-Verlag, New York, 60-78.

Druckrey H., Preussmann R., Ivankovic S., and Schmähl D. (1967). Organotrope carcinogene Wirkungen bei 65 verschiedenen N-Nitroso-Verbindungen an BD-Ratten. Z. Krebsforsch., 69, 103-201.

Ehrenberg L. and Holmberg B. (1978). Extrapolation of carcinogenic risk from animal experiments to man. Env. Health Persp., 22, 33-35.

Englund A. and Holmberg B. (1976). Recent achievements and research initiated in the Swedish plastics and rubber industry. Environm. Hlth Persp., 17, 237-239.

Hammond E.C., Selikoff I.J., Lawther P.L., and Seidman H. (1976). Inhalation of benzpyrene and cancer in man. Ann. N.Y. Acad. Sci., 271, 116-124.

Holmberg B., Kronevi T. and Winell M. (1976). The pathology of vinyl chloride exposed mice. Acta vet. scand., 17, 328-342.

Holmberg B. and Sjöström B. (1977). Toxicological review on rubber chemicals. Investigation Report 1977:19, National Board of Occupational Safety and Health, Stockholm, 1-100.

Holmberg B. and Westlin A. (1978). Considerations in the decision of the Swedish occupational standard for VCM. Ann. N.Y. Acad. Sci., in press.

Horton A.W. and Denman D.T. (1955). Carcinogenesis of the skin. A re-examination of methods for the quantitative measurement of the potencies of complex materials. Cancer Res., 15, 701-709.

Hygieniska gränsvärden (1978) arbetarskyddsstyrelsen anvisningar nr 100, arbetarskyddsstyrelsen, Stockholm. English translation available.

Jones H.B. and Grendon A. (1975). Environmental factors in the origin of cancer and estimation of the possible hazard to man. Food Cosmet. Toxicol., 13, 251-268.

National Cancer Institute (1976). Guidelines for carcinogen bioassay of trichloroethylene. NCI Carcinogenesis, Technical Report Series No 2 DHEW Publ. No (NIH) 76-801, Washington D.C.

Olsson S. (1977). Proposal for the elimination of chemical hazards in the rubber
    industry. Investigation Report 1977:19, National Board of Occupational Safety
    and Health, Stockholm, 103-119.
Ott M.G., Holder B.B. and Gordon H.L. (1974). Respiratory cancer and occupational
    exposure to arsenicals. Arch. Environm. Health, 29, 250-255.
Payne W.W. and Hueper W.C. (1960). The carcinogenic effects of single and repeated
    doses of 3,4-benzpyrene. Am. Ind. Hyg. Ass. J., 21, 350-355.
Peto J. (1978). The hygiene standard for chrysotile asbestos. Lancet, March 4,
    484-489.
Poel E. (1956). Cocarcinogens and minimal carcinogenic doses. Science, 123, 588-
    589.
Preussmann R. (1976). Chemical carcinogens in the human environment - problems
    and quantitative aspects. Oncology, 33, 51-57.
Report of a Task Group (1978). Air pollution and cancer: risk assessment method-
    ology and epidemiological evidence. Env. Health Persp., 22, 1-12.
Saffiotti U. (1977). Scientific bases of environmental carcinogenesis and cancer
    prevention: developing an interdisciplinary science and facing its ethical
    implications. J. Tox. Env. Health, 2, 1435-1447.
Saffiotti U. (1978). Experimental identification of chemical carcinogens, risk
    evaluation, and animal to human correlations. Env. Health Persp., 22, 107-113.
Schmähl D., Port R. and Wahrendorf J. (1977). A dose-response study on urethane
    carcinogenesis in rats and mice. Int. J. Cancer, 19, 77-80.
Schneiderman M.A., Mantel N. and Brown C.C. (1975). From mouse to man or how to
    get from the laboratory to Park Avenue and 59th street. Ann. N.Y. Acad. Sci.,
    246, 237-248.
Selikoff I.J. (1975). Recent perspectives in occupational cancer. Ambio, 4, 14-17.
Säfwenberg J.-O. and Holmberg B. (1975). Kvalitativa och kvantitativa aspekter på
    kemisk carcinogenes. Undersökningsrapport AMMT 103/75, arbetarskyddsstyrelsen,
    Stockholm.
Weinberg A.M. (1972). Science and trans-science. Minerva, 10, 209-222.
Wettström R. and Zetterkvist E. (1978). Personal communication.
Williams M.H.C. (1958). Occupational tumors of the bladder. In: R.W. Raven (Ed.)
    Cancer Vol 3, Butterworth, London, 337-380.
Zbinden G. (1978). Progress in toxicology. Special topics. Vol. 1. Springer-Verlag,
    New York, 1973, 18.

Seroepidemiology and Human Cancer

Seroepidemiology of the Epstein-Barr Virus and Its Causative Role in Human Tumours

Guy de-Thé*

International Agency for Research on Cancer, Lyon, France

INTRODUCTION

Three complementary approaches have been developed in cancer research. The first was the experimental approach in animals where both spontaneous tumours and experimental inoculations of substances believed to be associated with human cancer were studied. The second approach has been an extensive search for the understand- of the basic mechanisms which enable a normal cell to become malignant and to escape the normal host control for its growth. Oncogenic viruses remain unique tools for such studies. although they do not yet permit the elucidation of the pathogenesis of cancer at the cellular level. A third and, up to now, least developed approach has been the direct study of human tumours using epidemiological tools. The case of the Epstein-Barr virus (EBV) represents a model where epidemiological studies, well integrated with laboratory investigation, permits a start to the understanding of the role of the virus in human malignancies.

The Epstein-Barr virus, a new human herpesvirus, isolated from a tumour biopsy of a child with Burkitt's lymphoma (Epstein, Achong and Barr, 1964), is a widely spread agent, present in all ethnic groups and geographical areas. How can such a widely spread agent be responsible for Burkitt's lymphoma (BL), arising in very limited geographical areas, or for nasopharyngeal carcinoma (NPC), restricted to certain ethnic groups ? This dilemma is probably the reason why the Epstein-Barr virus has been, since the date of its discovery, the "mal-aimé" of viral oncology. It is fascinating then, to see that this virus represents, today, the first established oncogenic agent in the human species.

We shall review how seroepidemiology was instrumental in assessing the role of this virus in infectious mononucleosis (IM), in Burkitt's lymphoma (BL) and in naso-pharyngeal carcinoma (NPC). We shall also assess, for the future, the value of the seroepidemiological approach for the control of these diseases.

---

* On leave to the Department of the Regius Professor of Medicine - ICRF - Cancer Epidemiology Unit - University of Oxford, England.

THE AGE OF INFECTION, AND POSSIBLY THE STRAIN OF EBV VARY AROUND THE
WORLD.

Henle was the first to show the ubiquity of the infection by EBV and the critical
role of socio-economic level in the age specific prevalence of EBV infection
(which reflects the age of primary infection, since antibodies to the EBV structural
antigen (VCA) are quite stable) (Henle and others, 1969). Henle observed that
children living in the "slums" of the US towns were infected much earlier than
those living in high class areas. We extended these studies in investigating
representative samples of the general population in Uganda, Singapore, Hong Kong
and the East of France. As seen in Fig. 1, we observed highly significant
differences in the age of primary infection by EBV, and in the immune response to
both VCA and EA antigens, between areas of high incidence for Burkitt's lymphoma
(Uganda), or for nasopharyngeal carcinoma (Singapore, Hong Kong) (de-Thé and others,
1975 a). These data suggested to us that, in contrast with the situation of infectious mononucleosis, where a delayed primary EBV infection is the critical factor
for EBV to induce the disease, a very early infection, possibly in the perinatal
period of life, might represent the extreme condition necessary for Burkitt's
lymphoma development (de-Thé, 1977).

The mode of infection is probably critical in the pathogenesis of EBV-associated
diseases. For infectious mononucleosis, it is believed that the virus is transmitted by saliva, hence the role of deep kissing between a susceptible EBV-negative
adolescent and an EBV-shedder. The mode of infection of babies in Equatorial
Africa is unknown, but saliva again could play a critical role. The habit of kiss-
feeding remains widely spread among the mothers and more than 50% of the adults
are EBV-shedders in their saliva. Exchange of saliva between the mother and the
new-born could well be a source of heavy infection. Another possibility is
breast feeding, since the presence of EBV-infected lymphocytes in human milk has
been established (Feller and others, unpublished data).

Strain differences between EBV around the world is a subject of great interest in
many laboratories and although there are not yet clear-cut differences between
EBV isolates originating from different ethnic groups or diseases, molecular
virologists appear to be on the verge of finding differences in viral DNA sequences
between different strains of EBV.

NEED FOR CO-FACTORS

The development of a cancer represents a *multifactorial event* and until we understand the basic mechanisms of the mutation of a normal cell into a cancerous cell
we are left with the characterization of the more immediate causes of the diseases
to try and control them. Environmental factors are believed to cause around 80%
of all cancers (Doll, 1977) while host factors may play a role in modulating the
susceptibility of the individuals to specific environmental carcinogens. In the
field of EBV and human tumours, co-factors are essential for tumour development.
In Burkitt's lymphoma, the epidemiological characteristics of the tumour cannot
be explained by those of EBV infection, and the role of malaria has been stressed
since the early studies on BL (Dalldorf and others, 1964; Burkitt, 1969; O'Conor,
1970; IARC Annual Report, 1976, 1977). Malaria, being immuno-suppressive, could
help a clone of tumour cells to escape the central immune surveillance, but malaria
antigens being stimulators for B cells proliferation, could also increase the
number of target cells for EBV transformation (Greenwood and others, 1972).
Implication of malaria in BL causation must be more complex and an experimental
model system in which both EBV and malaria could be investigated is badly needed.

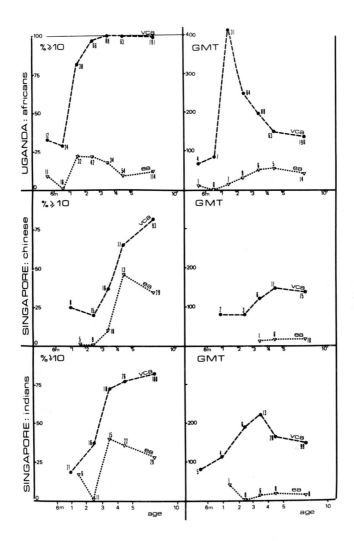

Fig. 1. Prevalence (curves at left) and geometric mean
titers (GMT of positive sera: curves at right)
of antibodies to VCA and EA in representative
samples of three populations: Ugandans (at high
risk for BL), Chinese Singaporeans (at high risk
for NPC) and Indian Singaporeans (at no risk for
BL or NPC).
The number of sera for each point of the curves are noted.
(Reproduction with permission from Lancet).

For nasopharyngeal carcinoma, chemical carcinogens in the environment as well as host genetic factors seem to play a critical role in the development of the tumour. Ho has repeatedly stressed the possible role of nitrosamines contained in unclean salted fish which represents a delicatessen for the Cantonese Chinese. Huang and co-workers (1978) have succeeded in inducing tumours of the nasal fossa in rats fed on salted fish and when one recalls the tissue tropisms of the nitrosamines for the ENT, it is certainly important to encourage studies in that direction. The point of the matter is that NPC is not, as we shall see below, only observed in Southern Chinese but also in many Arab countries and one will have to find the dietary habits of these populations which could favour the exposure of the future patients to nitrosamines contained in food or fumes. Clifford (1972) has stressed the role of fumes containing polycyclic aromatic hydrocarbons in the huts of East Africa and their possible association with the development of nasopharyngeal carcinoma. The role of genetic factors in NPC has been the subject of many studies and Simons and co-workers (1977) found that the HLA haplotype A2-B Sin-2 presented an increased relative risk by a factor of 2 in Cantonese Chinese.

Further studies on possible co-factors in EBV-associated tumours such as BL and NPC are of great importance because it might be easier to intervene against these co-factors than against the Epstein-Barr virus itself. The example of Burkitt's lymphoma for which an anti-malaria scheme has been implemented in the North Mara district of Tanzania by the IARC and the Tanzanian government in the Spring of 1978 is a relatively simple and beneficial action which may well prevent the disease. At the same time, such intervention should help in understanding the pathogenesis of the oncogenic activity of the EBV in these populations.

EBV AND INFECTIOUS MONONUCLEOSIS: *The critical role of the age of infection and of the host immune response.*

Henle and co-workers, in 1968, observed by chance a case of infectious mononucleosis in a laboratory assistant who lacked antibodies and sero-converted at the time of the illness. Then, Evans and co-workers (1968), who were following Yale University students entering college in the period of 1968-1973, found that lacking antibodies to EBV was a necessary condition for the development of infectious mononucleosis: among 268 college students entering university and lacking EBV antidodies, 15% developed infectious mononucleosis (IM) whereas among the 94 students who exhibited EBV antibodies, none developed clinical IM. They further showed that sero-conversion with EBV, correlated well with heterophile antibodies. Later on, many studies confirmed this original observation, indicating that EB virus is the cause of most of the IM syndromes.

Fig. 2 gives the typical EBV serological profile during the clinical course of IM. During the incubation period, IgM and IgG antibodies to the viral capsid antigens (VCA) develop, but one has to wait for the clinical phase of the disease, to see antibodies to early antigens (EA) arising. EA-D antibodies increase in titer up to the convalescent period where they decrease progressively to disappear after months to a year. In contrast, antibodies to the nuclear antigen (EBNA) are lacking during the acute phase of the disease and develop during the convalescence period sometimes after months to a year. This profile (increasing titers of antibodies to EA and VCA and absence of antibodies to EBNA) reflects a recent primary infection by the EBV. EBV is found in the throat washings of patients with infectious mononucleosis, for as long as six months and sometimes a year after accute illness (Chang and Golden, 1971; Miller and others, 1973). Epithelial cells appear to be involved in the replication of EBV either in the oropharynx or possibly in the parotid gland.

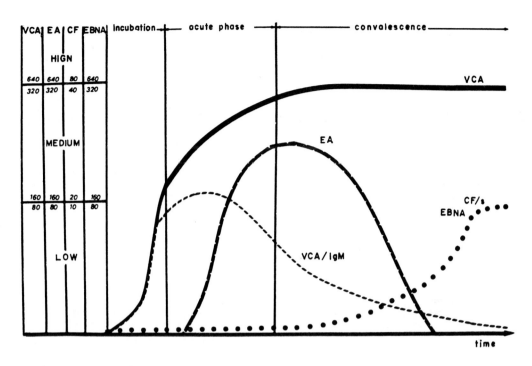

Fig. 2. EBV antibody response during the course of infectious mononucleosis.

EBV AND BURKITT'S LYMPHOMA: *We now have epidemiological evidence for a causal relationship between the EB virus and this tumour.*

Up to now, considerable circumstancial evidences supported a causal implication of EBV in the development of BL, but we now have epidemiological evidence that this is the case (de-Thé and others, 1978). The disease recognized by Burkitt in areas with minimal temperature of above 60°F and annual rainfall above 30 inches (Burkitt, 1959, 1962), and pathologically characterized by O'Conor and Davies (1960) is a lymphoma of children with peculiar geographical and age distribution.

Clinically, this tumour involves jaws, maxillaries, testis, ovaries but never the spleen nor the lymph nodes. This tumour was the first to show an excellent response to chemotherapy, first with cyclophosphamide, subsequently with vincristine methotrexate and cytosine arabinoside. Relapses occur very early in 50% of the cases, or if the first remission lasts at least 10 weeks, survival is excellent, involving about 75% of the children after five years (Ziegler, 1972).

The association between EBV and BL is based mainly on the seroepidemiological data comparing patients and various types of controls, and on the regular presence of EBV markers in the tumour cells (EBV/DNA and EBNA) (zur Hausen and others, 1970; Olweny and others, 1977). Henle and others (1969, 1970a, 1971) showed that BL patients regularly had higher antibody titers to VCA and to EA than various control groups (cancer patients, other diseases, and normal individuals). Antibodies directed against the early antigen (EA) type R (for restricted) were found to be of prognostic value (Henle and others, 1970b). This is of importance since antibodies to EA are the only antibodies to develop at the time of tumour onset (see below).

The knowledge of the EBV serological profile *prior* to the development of the
disease would, indeed, be critical in establishing the nature of the association
between EBV and this tumour, and would permit the characterixation of children at
highest risk of developing the tumour. In fact, this was the aim of the prospective study that we have carried out at IARC. This study, planned and discussed
between 1968 and 1970, was initiated in late 1971. The main hypothesis for the
study was to see if BL was developing in a situation similar to that of infectious
mononucleosis, namely that children lacking EBV antibodies were at high risk for
developing BL, or if, on the contrary, a long standing and heavy infection by EBV
was a favouring factor for the development of the tumour. Finally, one could test
prospectively a null hypothesis, i.e. that EBV was possibly a passenger virus,
infecting the tumour a posteriori.

The West Nile district of Uganda was selected as the study area since the incidence
of BL was high and the epidemiological characteristics of the tumour well documented. Feasibility studies were carried out in 1968 and 1969, and showed that antibodies to EBV structural antigen (VCA) were remarkably stable over 18 months time
and that 10% of the children had high titers (higher than 160) whereas 10% had low
titers (= 1-10). Assuming that either group might be the one from which children
will eventually develop BL with a 5 fold increased relative risk, then 30 cases of
Burkitt's lymphoma would be needed. It was estimated that 5 years follow up of
37 000 children, aged 4-8 should yield approximately that number of BL cases.

The organization of the survey took place during 1971 and in early 1972 the collection of blood from all the children in the four selected countries of the West Nile
district was initiated. In fact, by October 1974, serum samples had been obtained
from about 42 000 children aged 0-8. The search for all new cases of BL in the
survey population started in January 1973, with teams visiting regularly all health
centers, dispensaries and hospitals. By december 1977, 31 children had been
clinically diagnosed with BL in the study area, but only 14 originated from the
bled cohort. Fourteen is less than what was expected during a 5 years follow up
but it started before the whole population was bled and a decrease in the incidence
of BL was observed during the study period. In fact, the case detection is still
continuing and two new cases have been diagnosed in 1978, and this will carry on
for another year.

Antibodies to the various EBV antigens as well as antibodies against other herpesviruses were tested in the sera collected prior and after tumour development in
the 14 children but also in a number of controls of the same age, sex and locality.
Whereas no significant differences in titers were observed for antibody to EA or
to EBNA, significantly higher titers of antibody to VCA were observed in the pre-
BL sera when compared to various matched controls. The geometric mean titer for
BL patients was 425 in pre-BL sera versus 125 for the controls. When the titers
of the children who later on developed Burkitt's lymphoma were compared to random
samples of the population of the same age, the titers of all but 2 future BL cases
were higher than the mean of the corresponding age group of the normal population
(Fig. 3). An increased relative risk of 30 time was established for children
having VCA titers two dilutions or more above the mean standardized for age, sex
and locality. The above results establish EBV as a causative factor of BL.

However it is worth noting that 4 future BL cases did not have elevated EBV antibody
titers before the onset of the disease. One had clinical characteristics of a
lymphosarcoma but not of a BL type and exhibited antibodies to EA-D, atypical of BL.
Another case was diagnosed as a retinoblastoma or unclassified lymphoma and had no
EBV/DNA detectable in the tumour tissue. Whereas the remaining two cases had typical
clinical features of Burkitt's lymphoma, one lacked EBV/DNA in tumour tissue.

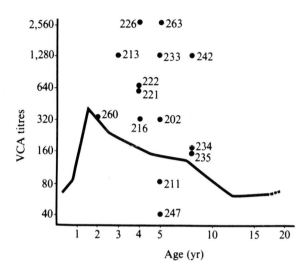

Fig. 3.   VCA antibody titres in sera collected from BL cases long before tumour
          manisfestation compared with mean antibody titers in random samples of
          the population of the study area. (black curve)

Thus a typical BL showed no association with EBV neither at the serological level,
nor at the viral level. This suggests that in tropical regions there are two types
of   lymphomas   with different etiologies. The EBV-associated lymphomas
have high VCA titers long before clinical onset of the disease and detectable viral
DNA and viral nuclear antigen in the tumour cell. The EBV-free lymphomas would not
differ from the general population with regard to their EBV profile prior to tumour
development and would lack EBV marker in the tumour cells. Of interest is the fact
that most chilhood lymphomas in temperate climates represent EBV-free lymphomas
when this is the exception in tropical areas (de-Thé and others, 1978). It is
quite clear from the results of this study that, whereas EBV is an essential factor
for lymphomas as described by Burkitt in Equatorial Africa, other factors are
essential for the clinical disease to develop. Burkitt's lymphoma, like all cancers,
represents a multifactorial event. We have two factors, at hand, an EBV infection,
most probably early in life, with relative risk of 30, and hyper-endemic malaria,
although it is not yet proven. Host factors may play a critical role in the
development of BL, but no solid data are available.

How to prevent this childhood cancer ? Epstein has been an advocate for the
development of a vaccine against EBV (Epstein, 1976). Important effort is made
towards this direction in the United Kingdom and, to a lesser extent, in the
United States. Once an experimental model is properly set up, and a vaccine
developed, then the seroepidemiological experience that we have established in the
field will be essential to test this vaccine on human populations. An EBV vaccine,
however, might be difficult to justify for Burkitt's lymphoma, although it would
represent the ultimate proof of the causative role of the virus in the tumour.

Nevertheless, a vaccine could be much more useful as an intervention mechanism to prevent a much more frequent tumour, namely nasopharyngeal carcinoma (see below). Other alternatives exist for BL: an intervention against malaria is an obvious choice and the IARC has implemented an intervention scheme in Tanzania where 70 000 children aged 0-10 are being subjected to chloroquine tablets, twice a month, to prevent clinical malaria. In following up this population and comparing it to a control one, where no intervention is taking place, it should be possible to estimate the importance of malaria as a co-factor to BL and to prevent the tumour. Another approach would be to follow the natural socio-economic development having a direct effect on perinatal events, it will delay primary infection by EBV and therefore eliminate the circumstances favouring an early EBV infection, thus possibly preventing BL development.

EBV AND NASOPHARYNGEAL CARCINOMA: *The association is so close that EBV serology can now be used clinically.*

Seroepidemiology has also been very instrumental in understanding the relationship between EBV and nasopharyngeal carcinoma (NPC). NPC is clinically, epidemiological-ly and pathologically very different from BL. This tumour, developing in the lymphoepithelium of the nasopharynx, is characterized by its lymphotropism, as it invades cervical lymph nodes so early that this predominates the clinical picture. Although this tumour was described originally as a lymphoepithelioma, it is now clear from ultrastructural studies that it is a carcinoma with a regular and important infiltration of lymphoid elements. Whereas BL is very sensitive to chemotherapy, NPC is resistant to drug, but sensitive to radiation therapy. Epidemiologically, three different levels of incidence can be described around the world as seen in Fig. 4. The high risk area is centered around the Kwantung province of the People's Republic of China and in the Cantonese Chinese establish-ments in South East Asia and America, with an incidence of 13 to 30 per 100 000 inhabitants. An intermediate area is spreading over North and East Africa and in some of the countries around the Mediterranean Sea, with an incidence of 1.2 to 9 per 100 000 inhabitants. In all the rest of the world, including Western Europe and the United States, the tumour is very rare, with an incidence lower than 1 per 100 000 inhabitants.

Seroepidemiology has shown a regular association, wherever in the world, between high antibody response to the various EBV determined antigens and the tumour, when compared with patients with other ENT tumours, other tumours and the normal popula-tion of the same area and ethnic group. In fact, as in BL, the association between EBV and NPC rests upon the antibody profile of the patients, and upon the regular presence of EBV markers in the epithelial tumour cells (Henle and others, 1970b ; zur Hausen and others, 1970; de-Thé and others, 1973; Klein and others, 1974; Huang and others, 1974; de-Thé and others, 1975b). Of particular interest is the fact that the EBV serology profile does develop well in parallel with the clinical evolution of the disease. Fig. 5 shows that the four EBV reactivities evolve in parallel with the clinical deterioration and that among the serological reactiv-ities, the titers of antibody to EA-D (for diffuse) show the greatest difference between patients with other tumours and controls even at stage 1 of the disease. Thus, EBV serology could now be used by the clinicians for helping in the diagnosis of NPC in the case of tumorous cervical lymphnodes adenopathies with unknown primary. EBV serology could also be used for assessing the prognosis of NPC. In a retrospective study, Henle and co-workers (1977) found that rising titers of EA-D could preceed clinical relapse and represent a warning signal. A prospective study is now being implemented in Paris and in other collaborative centers in order to assess prospectively the clinical value of the EBV serology and to verify the suggestion of Chan and others (1977) that high EA reactivity prior to treatment could be used as a marker for the prognosis of the disease.

INCIDENCE OF CANCER OF THE NASOPHARYNX   males

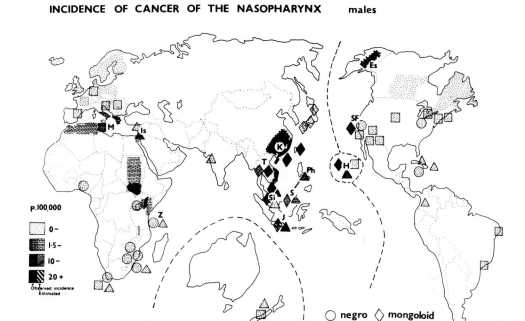

Fig. 4. World distribution of NPC.

Key   ES = Eskimos, H = Hawaii, Is = Israel, J = Java, K = Province of Kwantung
in the People's Republic of China, M = Malta, Ph = Philippines, S = Sumatra,
SF = San Francisco.

Geometric figures refer to Cancer Registries, whereas shaded areas refer to
estimated incidence from relative frequency data.   This map was kindly prepared by
Ms Paula Cook, Department of the Regius Professor of Medicine, University of Oxford,
England.

Also of great interest are the recent findings on IgA antibodies in sera and saliva
from NPC patients.   IgA antibody specific to EBV (VCA and EA) are greatly elevated
in sera of NPC patients (Henle and others, 1976).   Titers of IgA antibodies
fluctuate with the clinical evolution (Henle and others, 1977) and a prospective
follow up of NPC patients actually implemented at the Institut Gustave Roussy in
Paris and at collaborating institutes will determine the clinical usefulness of
such antibodies.   Secretory IgA specific for VCA and EA were observed by Desgranges
and others (1977a) in the *saliva* of NPC patients and up to now in other conditions.
Although IgA in saliva usually originates in parotide salivary glands, such IgA
were found in the tumour itself (Desgranges and others, 1977b).   Thus the search
for IgA specific for VCA and EA in saliva could be used for mass detection of the
tumour in high risk areas.

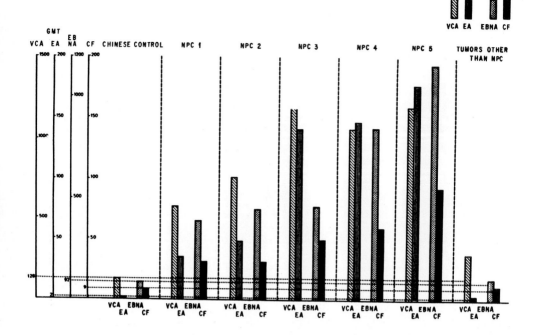

Fig. 5.   The evolution of the various EBV activities (EBNA, CF/s, VCA and EA) with
the clinical deterioration of NPC from stage 1 to stage 5 of the disease.
(Reproduction with permission from the Int. J. Cancer).

CONCLUSIONS   *Vaccine against EBV and future of EBV and human tumours.*

From the above one can conclude that seroepidemiology has been a key factor for the
understanding of the role of EBV in human diseases as this approach permitted to
discover that EBV was the cause of infectious mononucleosis and later on to provide
the first epidemiological evidence of a causal relationship between a virus and a
human cancer, namely Burkitt's lymphoma (de-Thé and others, 1978).

The second important value of seroepidemiology has been to understand the epidemiology of the infection by this virus and the relation between the age of infection
and the disease profile. We already knew from the studies of paralytic poliomyelitis
that the age of infection by a very common virus could be a determining factor for
causation of a specific disease. Again we now learn the lesson from EBV, infectious
mononucleosis and Burkitt's lymphoma where the age of the primary infection
determine the development of two widely differing diseases.

The third important value of seroepidemiology is to prepare for the eventual testing
of a vaccine. Epstein is very advanced in pushing ahead the idea and a program of
an EBV vaccine development. It is obvious that the future testing of a vaccine
could not be considered without the basic data obtained in the seroepidemiological
surveys of normal populations as conducted in Uganda and in the Far East. It is
out of the scope of this paper to discuss both the technical difficulties in
developing an EBV vaccine and the ethical problem to eventually test it. Infectious
mononucleosis is a minor disease and justification of a vaccine program could only
come from the increased risk for Hodgkin's disease observed for those who have had
infectious mononucleosis (Munoz and others, 1978). The prevention of Burkitt's

lymphoma has been discussed above and a vaccine could hardly be considered as a top priority by the African Ministry of Health. On the other hand an EBV vaccine could be of great interest in the prevention of nasopharyngeal carcinoma, provided that cell mediated immune processes play a critical role in tumour development in pre-clinical events. It is not our intention here to suggest that every Cantonese Chinese should be vaccinated at birth against EBV. However, if a prospective study could characterize better the highest risk group for this tumour, it would be ethically acceptable to try a protective vaccine in such individuals to be given prior the age of highest risk for the tumour.

Can our knowledge in EBV seroepidemiology be of practical use in medicine ? The answer is yes, and the clinical value of EBV serology in the management of NPC covers the diagnosis, the prognosis, and the prospects are good that it will be useful for managing the treatment of NPC.

REFERENCES

Burkitt, D. P. (1959). A sarcoma involving the jaws in African children. Brit. J. Surg., 46, 218-223.
Burkitt, D. P. (1962). A children's cancer development upon climatic factors. Nature (London), 194, 232-234.
Burkitt, D. P. (1969) Etiology of Burkitt's lymphoma. An alternative to a vectored virus. J. Natl. Cancer Inst., 42, 19-28.
Chan, S. H., de-Thé, G. and Goh, E. H. (1977). Prospective study of EBV antibody titers and survival in patients with nasopharyngeal carcinoma. Lancet, i, 948-949.
Chang, R. S. and Golden, H. D. (1971). Transformation of human leukocytes by throat washing from infectious mononucleosis patients. Nature (London), 234, 359-360.
Clifford, P. (1972). Carcinogens in the nose and throat: nasopharyngeal carcinoma in Kenya. Proc. Roy. Soc. Med., 65, 682-686.
Dalldorf, G., Linsell, C. A., Barnhart, F. E. and Martyn, F. (1964). An epidemiological approach to the lymphomas of African children and Burkitt's sarcoma of the jaws. Perp. Biol. Med., 7, 435-449.
Desgranges, C., de-Thé, G., Ho, J. H. C. and Ellouz, R. (1977a). Neutralizing EBV specific IgA in throat-washings of nasopharyngeal carcinoma (NPC) patients. Int. J. Cancer, 19, 627-633.
Desgranges, C., Li, J. Y. and de-Thé, G. (1977b). EBV specific secretory IgA in saliva of NPC patients. Presence of secretory piece in epithelial malignant cells. Int. J. Cancer, 20, 881-886.
de-Thé, G. (1977). Is Burkitt's lymphoma (BL) related to a perinatal infection by Epstein-Barr virus (EBV)? Lancet, i, 335-338.
de-Thé, G., Ablashi, D. V., Liabeuf, A. and Mourali, N. (1973). Nasopharyngeal Carcinoma VI. Presence of an EBV specific nuclear antigen in fresh tumour biopsies. Preliminary results. Biomedicine, 19, 349-352.
de-Thé, G., Day, N. E., Geser, A., Lavoué, M-F., Ho, J. H. C., Simons, M. J., Sohier, R., Tukei, P., Vonka, V. and Zavadova, H. (1975a). Seroepidemiology of the Epstein-Barr virus - Preliminary analysis of an international study. In G. de-Thé, M. A. Epstein and H. zur Hausen (Eds.), Oncogenesis and Herpesviruses II, Lyon, International Agency for Research on Cancer, Sci. Publ. 11, Vol. 2, pp. 3-16.

de-Thé, G., Geser, A., Day, N. E., Tukei, P. M., Williams, E. H., Beri, D. P., Smith, P. G., Dean, A. G., Bornkamm, G. W., Feorino, P., Henle, W. (1978). Epidemiological evidence for causal relationship between Epstein-Barr virus Burkitt's lymphoma from Ugandan prospective study. Nature, 274, 756-761.

de-Thé, G., Ho, J. H. C., Ablashi, D. V., Day, N. E., Macario, A. J. L., Martin-Berthelon, M-C., Pearson, G. and Sohier, R. (1975). Nasopharyngeal Carcinoma IX. Antibodies to EBNA and correlation with response to other EBV antigens in Chinese patients. Int. J. Cancer, 16, 713-721.

Doll, R. (1977). Strategy for detection of cancer hazards to man. Nature, 265, 589-596.

Epstein, M. A. (1976). Implications for a vaccine for the prevention of Epstein-Barr virus infection: ethical and logistic considerations. Cancer Res., 36, 711-714.

Epstein, M. A., Achong, B. G. and Barr, Y. M. (1964). Virus particules in cultured lymphoblasts from Burkitt's lymphoma. Lancet, i, 702-703.

Evans, A. S., Niederman, J. C. and McCollum, R. W. (1978). Sero-epidemiologic studies of infectious mononucleosis with EB virus. New Engl. J. Med., 279, 1121-1127.

Greenwood, B. M., Bradley-Moore, A. M., Palit, A. and Brycesson, A. D. M. (1972). Immuno-suppression in children with malaria. Lancet, i, 169-172.

Henle, G., Henle, W. and Diehl, V. (1968). Relationship of Burkitt's tumour associated herpes type virus to infectious mononucleosis. Proc. Natl. Acad. Sci. USA, 59, 94-101.

Henle, G., Henle, W., Klein, G., Gunven, P., Clifford, P., Morrow, R. H. and Ziegler, J. L. (1971). Antibodies to early Epstein-Barr virus-induced antigens in Burkitt's lymphoma. J. Natl. Cancer Inst., 46, 861-871.

Henle, G. and Henle, W. (1976). Epstein-Barr virus-specific IgA serum antibodies as an outstanding feature of nasopharyngeal carcinoma. Int. J. Cancer, 17, 1-7.

Henle, W., Henle, G., Burtin, P., Cachin, Y., Clifford, P., De Schryver, A., de-Thé, G., Diehl, V., Ho, H. C. and Klein, G. (1970a). Antibodies to Epstein-Barr virus in nasopharyngeal carcinoma, other head and neck neoplasms and control groups. J. Natl. Cancer Inst., 44, 225-231.

Henle, W., Henle, G., Zajac, B., Pearson, G., Waubke, R. and Scriba, M. (1970b). Differential activity of human sera with early antigens induced by Epstein-Barr virus. Science, 169, 188-190.

Henle, W., Ho, J. H. C., Henle, G., Chan, J. C. W. and Kwan, H. C. (1977). Nasopharyngeal carcinoma: significance of changes in Epstein-Barr related antibody patterns following therapy. Int. J. Cancer, 20, 663-672.

Huang, D. P., Ho, J. H. C., Henle, W. and Henle, G. (1974). Demonstration of Epstein-Barr virus-associated nuclear antigen in nasopharyngeal carcinoma cells from fresh biopsies. Int. J. Cancer, 14, 580-588.

Huang, D. P., Ho, J. H. C., Saw, D. and Teoh, T. B. (1978). Carcinoma of the nasal and paranasal regions in rats fed Cantonese salted marine fish. In G. de-Thé and Y. Ito (Eds.). Nasopharyngeal Carcinoma: Etiology and Control, Lyon, International Agency for Research on Cancer, Sci. Publ. 20, pp. 315-328.

IARC Annual Reports (1976, 1977). International Agency for Research on Cancer, Lyon, France.

Klein, G., Giovanella, B. C., Lindahl, T., Fialkow, P. J., Singh, S. and Stehlin, J. (1974). Direct evidence for the presence of Epstein-Barr virus DNA and nuclear antigen in malignant epithelial cells from patients with anaplastic carcinoma of the nasopharynx. Proc. Natl. Acad. Sci. USA, 71, 4737-4741.

Miller, G., Niederman, J. C. and Andrews, L. (1973). Prolonged oropharyngeal excretion of Epstein-Barr virus after infectious mononucleosis. New Engl. J. Med., 288, 229-232.

Munoz, N., Davidson, R. J. L., Witthoff, B., Ericson, J. E. and de-Thé, G. (1978). Infectious mononucleosis and Hodgkin's disease. Int. J. Cancer, 22, 10-13.

O'Conor, G. T. (1970). Persistent immunology stimulation as a factor in oncogenesis with special reference to Burkitt's tumour. Am. J. Med., 48, 279-285.

O'Conor, G. T. and Davies, J. N. P. (1963). Malignant tumours in African children with reference to malignant lymphoma. Trop. J. Pediat., 56, 526-535.

Simons, M. J., Wee, G. B., Singh, D., Dharmalingham, S., Yong, N. K., Chau, J. C. W., Ho, J. H. C., Day, N. E. and de-Thé, G. (1977). Immunogenetic aspects of nasopharyngeal carcinoma. V. Confirmation of a Chinese related HLA profile (A2, Singapore 2) associated with an increased risk in Chinese for NPC. In "Epidemiology and Cancer Registries in the Pacific", NCI Monograph 47, pp. 147-151.

Ziegler, J. L. (1972). Chemotherapy of Burkitt's lymphoma. Cancer, 30, 1534-1540.

zur Hausen, G., Schulte-Holthausen, H., Klein, G., Henle, W., Henle, G., Clifford, P. and Santesson, L. (1970). EBV DNA in biopsies of Burkitt's tumours and anaplastic carcinomas of the nasopharynx. Nature (London), 228, 1056-1058.

Sero-epidemiology of Primate Herpesviruses and Associated Tumors as Models for Human Tumors

Lawrence A. Falk, Jr.

Departments of Microbiology, Rush-Presbyterian-St. Luke's and University of Illinois Medical Centers, Chicago, Illinois 60612, U.S.A.

ABSTRACT

The Epstein-Barr virus (EBV) of man is a B-lymphotropic herpesvirus which is ubiquitous in the population and most individuals show no clinical manifestations after primary infection. Some individuals who acquire EBV infection during adolescence develop heterophile-positive infectious mononucleosis. Furthermore, EBV has been shown to be associated with Burkitt's lymphoma and nasopharyngeal carcinoma. Certain B- and T-lymphotropic herpesviruses of Old and New World monkeys offer good models for studying the putative association of herpesviruses with human neoplasia. Herpesvirus papio, a B-lymphotropic virus of baboons and Herpesvirus saimiri, a T-lymphotropic herpesvirus of squirrel monkeys are of interest because these viruses apparently cause no disease in the natural hosts but can induce a spectrum of lymphoproliferative diseases in marmoset monkeys.

Key words: Epstein-Barr virus, Herpesvirus papio, Herpesvirus saimiri, Herpesvirus ateles, lymphotropic herpesviruses, lymphoproliferative disease, lymphoblastoid cells, latent infection, B-lymphocytes, T-lymphocytes, lymphocyte transformation

INTRODUCTION

Members of the herpesvirus group appear to possess a unique property: once the natural host becomes infected, infection persists for life. Throughout life, latent infections may be 1) completely inapparent without clinical disease, 2) recurrent disease at periodic intervals or 3) oncogenic as has been suggested for some herpesviruses. Representative human and primate herpesviruses (Fig. 1) are classified on the basis of the tissue in which they exist in a repressed state: neurotropic or lymphotropic. The neurotropic group is exemplified by herpes simplex virus types I and II which are harbored repressed in cells of the trigeminal or sacral ganglia respectively. The lymphotropic viruses are further subdivided into B- or T-tropic on the basis of the lymphocyte population they infect and transform in vivo or in vitro. EBV of man is the best known member of this group but recently viruses have been identified in Old World primates--specifically Herpesvirus papio of baboons (Falk and colleagues, 1976; Rabin and colleagues, 1977; Gerber and colleagues, 1977), viruses of chimpanzees (Gerber, Pritchett and Kieff, 1976) and orang-utans (Rasheed and colleagues, 1977). By the fact that gorillas and gibbon apes also have antibodies cross-reacting with EBV viral capsid antigens makes it reasonable to predict that these primates also have their own

HUMAN-PRIMATE HERPESVIRUSES

NEUROTROPIC	LYMPHOTROPIC	
	T-	B-
HERPES SIMPLEX I & II	HERPESVIRUS SAIMIRI	EPSTEIN-BARR VIRUS
VARICELLA-ZOSTER	HERPESVIRUS ATELES	HERPESVIRUS PAPIO
		CHIMPANZEE-VIRUS
		ORANG-UTAN VIRUS
		(GORILLA, GIBBON)

Fig. 1. Representative human and primate herpesviruses.

B-lymphotropic herpesviruses. All of these viruses possess cross-reacting viral capsid antigens with EBV and partial genome homology with EBV DNA.

Two T-lymphotropic herpesviruses have been identified in primates: Herpesvirus saimiri (HVS) of squirrel monkeys (Melendez and associates, 1968) and Herpesvirus ateles (HVA) of spider monkeys (Melendez and colleagues, 1972; Falk and colleagues, 1974). There appears to be a distinct division: B-tropic herpesviruses have thus far been identified only in man and Old World primate species and the T-lymphotropic viruses appear restricted to New World primates. One can ask the question whether T-viruses exist in man or Old World primates or if New World monkeys have B-tropic viruses. This of course is a possibility but on the basis of serologic studies we have performed, such viruses must be unrelated to these agents for man and Old World primates lack antibodies reactive against HVS or HVA and New World monkeys lack anti-EBV antibodies.

The etiologic association of EBV with heterophile-positive infectious mononucleosis and the possible cocarcinogenic role of EBV in Burkitt's lymphoma make the lymphotropic herpesviruses of nonhuman primates of interest as laboratory models for investigating the role of EBV in lymphoproliferative diseases of man. In the last decade, laboratories have employed nonhuman primate models for examining the oncogenic potential of lymphotropic herpesviruses. Herpesvirus papio of baboons and Herpesvirus saimiri of squirrel monkeys are good models for studying both viral induced malignancies or persistent, latent infections because it is possible to study latent infections in the natural hosts, baboons or squirrel monkeys respectively, or induce experimentally, malignancies or latent infections in marmoset monkeys (Saguinus, Callithrix sp.). Summarized herein are studies with Herpesvirus papio and Herpesvirus saimiri performed in the author's laboratory in collaboration with other investigators.

TABLE 1   Properties of Baboon Lymphoblastoid Cell lines Carrying <u>Herpesvirus</u> <u>papio</u>

	Baboon species	
	<u>P</u>. hamadryas	<u>P</u>. anubis
Origin of cell cultures	splenic lymphocytes	circulating lympho-cytes
LCL established	3	13
VCA/EA reactive cells	2/3[1] (2-10%)[2]	11/11 (1-10%)
EBNA-NA reactive cells	0/3	0/11
EBV-related genomes	3/3 (1-6)[3]	7/7 (12-25)
Rosette formation:		
E	0/3	0/8
EAC	3/3 (15-90%)	4/6 (2-7%)
Ig Production		
IgG	0/3	0/8
IgM	2/3 (21-24%)	8/8 (18-39%)

[1] Number positive/number tested
[2] Per cent positive cells: 200-300 cells examined in each test
[3] EBV-related genome equivalents per cell: EBV specific complementary RNA used in DNA-cRNA filter hybridization tests.

HERPESVIRUS PAPIO

Properties of Baboon Lymphoblastoid Cell Lines

Lymphoblastoid cell lines (LCL) were established from splenic or circulating lymphocytes of <u>Papio</u> <u>hamadryas</u> or <u>P</u>. <u>anubis</u> baboons (Table 1). With exception of one cell line, all cultures contained antigen-reactive cells that reacted with antibodies to EBV viral capsid or early antigens (VCA/EA). A nuclear antigen, similar or analogous to EBV specified nuclear antigen (EBNA) cannot be detected in cells of these cultures by immunofluorescence staining <u>in situ</u> with VCA+ human or baboon sera. A nuclear antigen has been detected in cells of some of these cultures by an acid-fixed nuclear binding technique (Ohno and associates, 1977).

Experimental Studies with Marmoset Monkeys

<u>Transformation of marmoset lymphocytes</u>. Lymphocytes of cotton-topped (CT) (<u>Saguinus oedipus</u>) or white-lipped (WL) (<u>S</u>. <u>nigricollis</u>, <u>S</u>. <u>fuscicollis</u>) marmosets were transformed <u>in vitro</u> after cocultivation with X-irradiated HVP-producing baboon lymphoblastoid cells (Falk and associates, 1977). The majority of CT LCL contained VCA/EA reactive cells, but all WL LCL were antigen-negative. EBNA-NA was not detected in any HVP-transformed marmoset LCL.

<u>Experimental inoculation of marmosets with HVP</u>. Three of 4 adult CT marmosets developed generalized lymphoproliferative disease and died 13-22 days postinoculation (PI) with 10^8 HVP-producing baboon lymphoblastoid cells (Table 2)

TABLE 2   Inoculation of adult CT or WL marmosets with HVP-producing baboon lymphoblastoid cells

Marmoset species	Animal number	Inoculum dose of cells (x 10^8)	VCA antibodies	Survival PI (days)
CT	KZ-1	1.3		17: generalized lymphoprolifera- tive disease
	DF-3	5.0	19[1]	22 "
	5833	5.0		13 "
	4472	5.0		550
WL	5471	5.0	16	550
	4261	5.0	16	550

[1]Day PI when VCA antibodies first detected in plasma of marmoset

(Deinhardt and colleagues, 1977). At necropsy, necrotic tumors were present at
the inoculation site and in addition pronounced hepatosplenomegaly and generalized
lymphadenopathy were found. Lymphoid hyperplasia was the prominent microscopic
lesion observed in spleen, lymph nodes, tonsils and thymus. Mild infiltration of
lymphoid cells was detected in liver, heart, lung, kidney and adrenal glands.

In contrast to the apparent susceptibility of adult CT marmosets to HVP infection,
experimental inoculation of newborn marmosets with HVP-producing cells resulted in
no overt clinical manifestations. In order to assess whether or not such marmosets
might respond differently when inoculated as adults, the marmosets described above
were re-inoculated with HVP-producing cells about 18 months after their first
inoculation. None of the animals developed a recognizable clinical illness after
the second inoculation and 3 of 4 reinoculated marmosets developed anti-HVP antibodies 10-24 days PI at titers ranging from 1:4 - 1:32. Additional evidence indicating HVP infection of these marmosets after the second inoculation comes from
the ability to establish continuous lymphoblastoid cell lines after cultivation
in vitro of their circulating lymphocytes. Continuous cell cultures were
established from lymphocytes of 4 re-inoculated marmosets. Preliminary
characterization of these cultures indicated they possessed a marmoset karyotype,
were antigen negative and had surface membrane properties of B-lymphocytes.

HERPESVIRUS SAIMIRI

Herpesvirus saimiri (HVS) and Herpesvirus ateles (HVA), in contrast to the
lymphotropic herpesviruses of Old World primates, show a specific tropism for
T-lymphocytes. This property makes HVS and HVA of interest because it provides a
model for studying the interaction of herpesviruses with T-lymphocytes and also it
is possible to establish continuous, T-lymphoblastoid cell lines from either
experimentally-induced tumors or after transformation in vitro of marmoset lymphocytes with HVA as described by Falk and colleagues (1974).

HVS in the Natural Host, Squirrel Monkeys

HVS was isolated originally by Melendez and his colleagues (1968) from kidney cell cultures of clinically-well squirrel monkeys (<u>Saimiri sciureus</u>) and was shown to be oncogenic for several species of New World monkeys. Subsequently Falk, Wolfe and Deinhardt (1972a, 1972b) studied the incidence of HVS infection in several colonies of squirrel monkeys using virus rescue and serologic techniques. These studies, summarized in Tables 3 and 4, showed that HVS was carried repressed in squirrel monkey lymphocytes, as HVS was recovered after lymphocytes or whole blood were cocultivated with permissive monolayer cells e.g. vero cells. Correlation of frequency of virus rescue with age of the monkeys indicated that as with herpes-virus infections in other animal species, the monkeys were born free of infection and acquired infection generally during their first year of life. As shown by virus isolation data presented in Table 3, HVS was rescued from 40% of lymphocyte preparations of squirrel monkeys ≤ 1 year of age in contrast to 80-91% recovery from lymphocytes of monkeys 2-3 years old. That HVS is carried repressed in squirrel monkey T-lymphocytes was demonstrated by Wright and colleagues (1976).

TABLE 3 Rescue of HVS from a colony of Squirrel Monkeys

Age group	Virus rescue		
	Total	Lymphocytes	Whole Blood
2 months	0/5[1]		0/5
≤ 1 year	7/16 (44)[2]	6/15 (40)	3/16 (19)
≥ 2 years	8/19 (42)	4/5 (80)	7/19 (37)
≥ 3 years	33/67 (49)	10/11 (91)	24/67 (36)
Total	48/107 (45)	20/31 (65)	34/107 (32)

[1] Number of monkeys positive/number monkeys tested
[2] percent positive monkeys

Examination of plasma, from squirrel monkeys used for virus rescue studies describ-ed above, for HVS specified antibodies, showed an excellent correlation between the two evaluation methods. As shown in Table 4, all monkeys about 2 months old and 10 of 16 monkeys one year of age lacked detectable antibodies to HVS as assayed by indirect immunofluorescence tests.

HVS infection amongst squirrel monkeys is probably initiated by oropharyngeal transmission as Falk and associates (1973) made repeated HVS isolation from oropharyngeal sections of 9 of 10 recently imported squirrel monkeys. HVS infection in these monkeys was confirmed by virus rescue and serologic assays.

Attempts to induce experimentally, a clinical disease after HVS inoculation of HVS seronegative, colony born/reared squirrel monkeys, yielded negative results (Falk, Wolfe and Deinhardt, 1973). The experimentally inoculated monkeys became infected and transmitted virus infection to their uninoculated cagemates but they have remained free of clinical disease for over six years' observation.

Comparison of Oncogenic and Attenuated Strains of HVS in Marmoset Monkeys

Several years ago an attenuated strain of HVS (A-HVS) was derived (Schaffer, Falk

TABLE 4 Plasma Antibodies to HVS Specified Late Antigens in a Colony of Squirrel
Monkeys

Age group	Number of monkeys	Number with HVS antibody titer[1]			
		≤4	4-16	32-64	128
2 months	2	2			
≤ 1 year	16	10	4	2	
≥ 2 years	19		12	5	2
≥ 3 years	67		13	48	6

[1]Reciprocal of plasma dilution giving positive staining in indirect immunofluorescence assays.

and Deinhardt, 1975) and opposed to oncogenic HVS (O-HVS) which is invariably
fatal in marmosets, marmosets inoculated with A-HVS became latently-infected but
remained free of fatal lymphoproliferative disease. Comparative properties of
O-HVS and A-HVS infection of marmoset monkeys are summarized in Table 5. O-HVS
causes malignant lymphoma-lymphocytic leukemia in marmoset monkeys. The mortality
rate is 100% once infection has been demonstrated by virus rescue and/or serologic
methods; as few as 2 plaque forming units (PFU) of HVS will cause lymphoma in CT
marmosets whereas 20 PFU of virus is required for infection of WL marmosets. The
survival period PI varies from 1-4 months and horizontal transmission of infection
to uninoculated cagemates apparently does not occur.

TABLE 5 Comparative Features of Experimental Infection of Marmoset Monkeys with
(Saguinus callithrix sp.) oncogenic or attenuated HVS

Clinical Disease	Lymphoma-Lymphocytic Leukemia	Self-limiting Lymphoproliferative Disease
Mortality rate:	100%	0%
Survival	1-4 months PI	4 years
Horizontal Transmission	No	No
Target Cells	T-lymphocyte	T-lymphocyte
Virus Expression in Target cell in vivo	Not detected	Not detected
Cultured in vitro	Viral antigen	Virus rescue
Antibody Response: Anti EA	Yes	Yes
Anti LA	Yes	Yes

In contrast, A-HVS induces only a self-limiting lymphoproliferative disease in
marmosets inoculated with virus doses ranging from 10^2 to 10^5 PFU. No marmosets
inoculated wtih A-HVS have ever died from causes which could be related to the

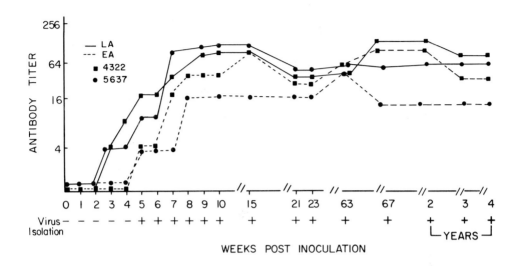

Fig. 2. Experimental infection of cotton-topped marmosets
with A-HVS: Virus rescue and antibody response.

virus inoculum. Shown in Fig. 2 is a longitudinal study with 2 cotton-topped
marmosets (animal number 4322 and 5637) which were inoculated with 600 PFU of
A-HVS over 4 years ago. A-HVS was rescued from both marmosets at 5 weeks PI after
cocultivation of their lymphocytes with Vero cells and it has been possible to
recover virus at all subsequent PI intervals. Semi-quantitation virus rescue
studies showed that 1-2 per 10^6 lymphocytes harbor HVS repressed. In addition
antibodies to HVS specified early and late antigens became detectable 2-4 weeks PI
and have persisted at relatively constant levels over the entire observation
period.

Although marmosets inoculated with A-HVS survive, recent studies we have performed
suggest a stage of lymphoproliferation 2-5 weeks PI based on semiquantitation virus
rescue (Wright and colleagues, 1979). Weekly assessment of the approximate number
of lymphocytes harboring HVS supressed in six inoculated common marmosets showed
that in all animals values increased from 3-85 at 2 weeks PI to 28-1,128 at 4
weeks PI and then declined to 2-270 by 12 weeks PI.

This observation implies that probably similar to marmosets infected with O-HVS,
HVS infection of target T-lymphocytes leads immediately to lymphoproliferation.
In marmosets infected with O-HVS, lymphoproliferation continues unabated until
death whereas in A-HVS infected marmosets, lymphoproliferation is abrogated 4-5
weeks PI and the infection resolves to a persistent, latent infection.

Are A-HVS latently infected marmosets resistant to challenge with O-HVS? The first
challenge studies reported by Schaffer, Falk and Deinhardt (1974) showed that
A-HVS infected cotton-topped marmosets, challenged with about 700 PFU of O-HVS,
survived 22 to 23 days PI compared to survival periods of 74 to 79 days for
marmosets without prior exposure to A-HVS. In more recent studies, Wright and
colleagues (1979), using A-HVS infected common marmosets described above, demonstrated that such animals resisted challenge with 100-850 PFU of O-HVS; these

challenged marmosets have now survived 1-2 years PI.

DISCUSSION

HVP and HVS are representative of B- and T-lymphotropic herpesviruses which in the natural hosts cause no overt clinical disease but in marmoset monkeys, HVP and HVS induce malignant or persistent, latent infections. The studies with HVP are relevant because of common properties shared with EBV: cross-reacting viral antigens, partial genome homology, transformation of lymphocytes in vitro and potential for inducing lymphoproliferative disease. In contrast, HVS/HVA are T-lymphotropic viruses: HVA transforms lymphocytes in vitro and both cause lymphoma in marmosets. The isolation of an attenuated strain of HVS, apparently lacking oncogenic potential, adds another approach for studying herpesvirus-induced malignancy/latent infections.

Until recently we have pursued these virus-host models for gaining insight into the oncogenic potential of herpesviruses to further support the assumption that EBV and herpes simplex virus cause neoplasia in man. While such studies are necessary and important, these models also present an excellent opportunity to study herpesvirus latency in the natural hosts, baboons and squirrel monkeys, and in an experimental host, marmoset monkeys. In the latter system we have some choice over the outcome of experimental infection: malignancy vs. persistent, latent infection. In the area of latent infections with lymphotropic herpes-viruses, our information is incomplete. Although we know these viruses are carried in either B- or T-lymphocytes, such lymphocytes have a definite lifespan and therefore there must be some means for perpetuating a given number of cells harboring repressed virus. This could be explained by at least one of two mechanisms: progenitor, hematopoietic stem cells harbor latent viral genomes which are passed to progeny cells or the infection is random and cyclic whereby a small percentage of infected lymphocytes are directed to enter the lytic cycle, infectious virus is produced which infects new lymphocytes.

Alternatively it is conceivable that a cell type other than lymphocytic cell harbor virus repressed and that lymphocytes are infected by virus released from such cells.

ACKNOWLEDGEMENTS

These studies were supported by Research Contract NO1-CP-33219 within the Virus Cancer Program of the National Cancer Institute, US Public Health Service and Research Grant VC-185 from the American Cancer Society. Lawrence Falk is a Scholar of the Leukemia Society of America, Inc. We thank the Board of Health, City of Chicago, for housing most of our experimental animals.

REFERENCES

Deinhardt, F., L. Falk, L. G. Wolfe, A. Schudel, M. Nonoyama, P. Lai, B. Lapin, and L. Yakovleva (1978). Susceptibility of marmosets to Epstein-Barr virus-like baboon herpesviruses. In E.I. Goldsmith and J. Moor-Jankowski (Eds.), Primates in Medicine, Vol. 10, S. Karger, Basel. pp. 163-170.
Falk, L. A., L. G. Wolfe, and F. Deinhardt (1972a). Isolation of Herpesvirus saimiri from blood of squirrel monkeys (Saimiri sciureus). J. Natl. Cancer Inst., 48, 1499-1505.
Falk, L., L. Wolfe, and F. Deinhardt (1972b). Epidemiology of Herpesvirus saimiri infection in squirrel monkeys. In E. I. Goldsmith and J. Moor-Jankowski (Eds.), Medical Primatology 1972, Part III, S. Karger, Basel. pp. 151-158.

Falk, L. A., S. Nigida, F. Deinhardt, R. W. Cooper, and J. I. Hernandez-Camacho (1973). Oral excretion of Herpesvirus saimiri in captive squirrel monkeys and incidence of infection in feral squirrel monkeys. J. Natl. Cancer Inst. 51, 1987-1989.

Falk, L. A., L. G. Wolfe, and F. Deinhardt (1973). Herpesvirus saimiri: Experimental infection of squirrel monkeys (Saimiri sciureus). J. Natl. Cancer Inst., 51, 165-170.

Falk, L. A., S. M. Nigida, F. Deinhardt, L. G. Wolfe, R. W. Cooper, and J. I. Hernandez-Camacho (1974). Herpesvirus ateles: properties of an oncogenic herpesvirus isolated from circulating lymphocytes of spider monkeys (Ateles sp.). Int. J. Cancer, 14, 473-482.

Falk, L., F. Deinhardt, M. Nonoyama, L. G. Wolfe, C. Bergholz, B. Lapin, L. Yakovleva, V. Agrba, G. Henle, and W. Henle (1976). Properties of a baboon lymphotropic herpesvirus related to Epstein-Barr virus. Int. J. Cancer, 18, 798-807.

Falk, L. A., G. Henle, W. Henle, F. Deinhardt, and A. Schudel (1977). Transformation of lymphocytes by Herpesvirus papio. Int. J. Cancer, 20, 219-226.

Gerber, P., R. F. Pritchett, and E. D. Kieff (1976). Antigens and DNA of a chimpanzee agent related to Epstein-Barr virus. J. Virol., 19, 1090-1099.

Gerber, P., S. S. Kalter, G. Schidlovsky, W. D. Peterson, Jr., and M. D. Daniel (1977). Biologic and antigenic characteristics of Epstein-Barr virus related herpesviruses of chimpanzees and baboons. Int. J. Cancer, 20, 448-459.

Melendez, L. V., M. D. Daniel, R. D. Hunt, and F. G. Garcia (1968). An apparently new herpesvirus from primary kidney cultures of the squirrel monkey (Saimiri sciureus). Lab. Anim. Care, 18, 374-381.

Melendez, L. V., R. D. Hunt, N. W. King, H. H. Barahona, M. D. Daniel, C. E. O. Fraser, and F. G. Garcia (1972). A new lymphoma virus of monkeys: Herpesvirus ateles. Nature New Biology, 234, 182-184.

Ohno, S., J. Luka, L. Falk, and G. Klein (1977). Detection of a nuclear, EBNA-type antigen in apparently EBNA-negative Herpesvirus papio (HVP)-transformed lymphoid lines by the acid-fixed nuclear binding technique. Int. J. Cancer, 20, 941-946.

Rabin, H., R. H. Neubauer, R. F. Hopkins, III, E. K. Dzhikidze, Z. V. Shevtsva, and B. A. Lapin (1977). Transforming activity and antigenicity of an Epstein-Barr-like virus from lymphoblastoid cell lines of baboons with lymphoid disease. Intervirology, 8, 240-249.

Rasheed, S., R. W. Rongey, J. Bruszweski, W. A. Nelson-Rees, H. Rabin, R. H. Neubauer, G. Esra, and M. B. Gardner (1977). Establishment of a cell line with associated Epstein-Barr-like virus from a leukemic orang-utan. Science, 198, 407-409.

Schaffer, P. A., L. A. Falk, and F. Deinhardt (1975). Brief Communication: Attenuation of Herpesvirus saimiri for marmosets after successive passage in cell culture at 39C. J. Natl. Cancer Inst., 55, 1243-1246.

Wright, J., L. A. Falk, D. Collins, and F. Deinhardt (1976). Mononuclear cell fraction carrying Herpesvirus saimiri in persistently infected squirrel monkeys. J. Natl. Cancer Inst., 57, 959-962.

Wright, J., L. A. Falk, L. G. Wolfe, J. Ogden, and F. Deinhardt (1977). Susceptibility of common marmosets (Callithrix jacchus) to oncogenic and attenuated strains of Herpesvirus saimiri. J. Natl. Cancer Inst., 59, 1475-1478.

Wright, J., L. A. Falk, L. G. Wolfe, and F. Deinhardt. Herpesvirus saimiri: Protective effect of attenuated strain against lymphoma induction. Submitted to J. Natl. Cancer Inst.

Seroepidemiology of Herpes Simplex Virus Type 2 and Cervical Carcinoma

W. E. Rawls

Department of Pathology, McMaster University, Hamilton, Ontario, Canada

ABSTRACT

A number of seroepidemiologic studies in which antibodies to herpes simplex virus type 2 (HSV-2) were measured in sera from women with neoplastic lesions of the cervix and control women have been undertaken. These studies have included assessment of neutralizing antibodies as a marker for past infections by the virus, quantitation of antibodies to virus-induced antigens in infected cells, correlations of antibody titers in terms of tumor burden and analysis of immunoglobulin class of antiviral antibody. In general, more antibodies to HSV-2 have been found among patients with preinvasive and invasive lesions of the cervix than among control women. However, considerable variability has been observed between the different studies. Much of this variability may be accounted for by the difficulties in accurately quantitating antibodies to HSV-2 in patients previously infected with HSV-1. While the data generated by the seroepidemologic studies support the hypothesis that HSV-2 is etiologically related to squamous cell carcinoma of the cervix, additional studies using more accurate antibody assay systems are needed to provide more convincing evidence.

INTRODUCTION

Analysis of sera for antibodies to viral antigens is an efficient method of assessing past infections by some viruses. In addition, antibody titers appear to correlate with the amounts of antigens to which the immune system of the patient has been exposed. Thus, seroepidemiological studies may entail both quantitative and qualitative estimates of antibodies to various viral antigens in an attempt to relate virus infections to disease states. A number of such studies have been undertaken in an attempt to relate herpes simplex virus type 2 (HSV-2) to squamous carcinoma of the cervix. The studies have included assaying for neutralizing antibodies in an effort to determine the occurrence of past infections by HSV-2 among cancer cases as compared to controls. Studies of the occurrence of antibodies to antigens expressed in cells but not incorporated into the virion have also been conducted as have studies in which antibody titers were correlated with tumor burden. Finally, a few

149

investigators have examined sera from cases of cervical cancer and from control women for antiviral antibody in certain immunoglobulin classes. The results of these studies have clearly demonstrated an association between HSV-2 and cervical cancer, however, the results have been variable. The purpose of this paper is to review the available data with respect to its conformity to the hypothesis that HSV-2 is etiologically related to the development of the cancer. This topic has been more extensively reviewed elsewhere (Aurelian and Strnad, 1976; Rapp and Reed, 1977; Rawls and Adam, 1977; Rawls et al., 1977; Melnick and Adam, 1978).

While herpes simplex virus type 2 (HSV-2) has unique biological, biochemical and epidemiological properties when compared to herpes simplex virus type 1 (HSV-1), the 2 viruses share cross-reacting antigens (Nahmias and Roizman, 1973). The genomes of both types of virus are relatively large and are capable of coding for multiple antigenic determinants. There is now abundant evidence indicating that the synthesis of the proteins coded for by the genomes is regulated; the proteins can be recognized as early (alpha proteins), intermediate (beta proteins) or late (gamma proteins) in relation to time after infection (Honess and Roizman, 1974). As a consequence antibodies with a variety of specificities are induced during virus infection. Some of these antibodies are directed against early proteins which are not represented on the virion, or minimally represented, while other antibodies are directed against late proteins which become structural components of the virus. Different assay techniques quantitate antibodies to different antigens and it is informative to consider the seroepidemiologic data with this in mind.

Neutralizing Antibodies

Since HSV-1 and HSV-2 share cross-reacting antigens, the concentrations of antibody to the two viruses have been measured and then the titers to the two viruses compared in most assays used to detect HSV-2 antibody. The values of the relative concentrations of antibody accepted as evidence for past infections with HSV-2 have been empirically derived. In comparing results from different studies, it was not possible to standardize for different criteria of positivity, thus, the information in this paper will generally be tabulated as reported in the literature.

Techniques based on measuring the rate of virus neutralization assess both the quality and the quantity of antibody. The results of 7 studies in which the kinetics of neutralization was used to measure antibodies in sera from women with invasive carcinoma and from control women are shown in Table 1. Significantly greater

TABLE 1   Antibodies to HSV-2 as Determined by Kinetics
of Neutralization

Percent with antibodies to HSV-2

Study area	Cases	Controls	References
Houston, Texas, USA	72	22	Rawls et al., 1969
Baltimore, Md. USA	100	67	Royston & Aurelian, 1970
Brussels, Belgium	83	33	Sprecher-Goldberger et al., 1970
Chicago, Ill., USA	48	18	Plummer & Masterson, 1971
Copenhagen, Den.	85	47	Vestegaard et al., 1972
Johannesburg, S.Africa	87	64	Freedman et al., 1974
Tokyo, Japan	75	71	Kawana et al., 1974

percents of women with cervical cancer had HSV-2 antibodies than
control women in all studies except for the study conducted in Tokyo,
Japan (Kawana et al., 1974).   More than 72% of the cancer cases were
found to have antibodies except for one study (Plummer and
Masterson, 1971).   The percent of control women with HSV-2 antibodies
varied from 18 to 71.

The results of neutralization kinetics have also been presented as
means instead of percent of patients positive by a specific criterion.
Skinner and coworkers (1971) found a mean K value of 0.96 for women
with invasive cancer and of 0.41 for control women.   These
differences were statistically significant as were the mean K values
0.65 and 0.49 found for cases and controls, respectively, by
Heyerdahl (1974).

A number of studies have been conducted in which antibody titers were
determined using a constant concentration of virus and varying
dilutions of sera.   The surviving virus was assayed after a constant
reaction time in cultures of cells grown in tubes or in microtiter
plates.   The results of assays in culture tubes are shown in Table
2.   Fifty percent or less of the women with cancer had antibodies to
HSV-2 by this assay and in all studies these percentages were more
than twice those observed in sera from control women.   The data

TABLE 2   Antibodies to HSV-2 as Determined by
Neutralization Assays

Percent with antibodies to HSV-2

Study area	Cases	Controls	References
Prague, Czechoslovakia	50	21	Janda et al., 1973
Tel Hashomer, Israel	15	7	Menczer et al., 1975
Pec, Hungary	50	9	Pasca et al., 1975
Turku, Finland	47	20	Peltonen, 1975

obtained in studies in which the surviving virus was assayed in
microtiter plates are summarized in Table 3.   It is apparent that
the occurrence of HSV-2 antibodies are greater among cancer cases
than among control women but the percentages positive for antibody
vary considerably between studies.

TABLE 3   Antibodies to HSV-2 as Determined by
Microneutralization

Percent Positive for HSV-2
Antibodies

Study area	Cases	Controls	References
Atlanta, Ga., USA	83	35	Nahmias et al., 1970
Auckland, New Zealand	31	23	Rawls, et al., 1970
Houston, Texas, USA	80[a] / 54[b]	52[d] / 23[b]	Adam et al., 1972
Yugoslavia	35[c] / 40[d]	23[c] / 25[d]	Kessler et al., 1974
Kampala, Uganda	81	71	Adam et al., 1974
Taipei, Taiwan	83[e]	23[e]	Kao et al., 1974
Montreal, Quebec	35	21	McDonald et al., 1974
Tegucigalpa, Honduras	68	46	Figueroa & Zambrana, 1976
Charleston, W.Virginia U.S.A.	45	17	Rawls & Adam, 1977
Osaka, Japan	28	15	Ozaki, et al., 1978

a.   Cases and controls predominantly black women
b.   Cases and controls predominantly white women
c.   Cases and controls predominantly Moslem
d.   Cases and controls predominantly non-Moslem
e.   Percent with titers to HSV-2 $\geq$ 1:16 considered positive

Antibodies Detected by Methods Other than Neutralization

The predomenance of antibodies among women with cervical cancer as
compared to women without the disease can also be demonstrated by
assays not involving neutralization. Examples of this are
illustrated in Table 4.

TABLE 4   Antibodies to HSV-2 as Assay on Fixed Cells
Infected with the Virus

Percent with Antibodies to HSV-2

Study area	Cases	Controls	References
Ibadan, Nigeria[a]	71	11	Adelusi et al., 1975
Cali, Colombia[b]	90	68	Munoz et al., 1975
Stockholm, Sweden[b]	81	27	Christensen & Espmark, 1976
Tokyo, Japan[c]	42	2	Ito et al., 1976

a.   Antibodies measured by indirect immunofluorescence

Table 3 continued.

b.   Antibodies measured by mixed hemadsorption
c.   Antibodies measured by anticomplement immunofluorescence

Cells infected with HSV-2 and fixed with acetone have been used as
a substrate to measure antibodies by indirect immunofluorescences
(Kao et al., 1974; Adelusi et al., 1975 and Munoz et al., 1975) and
by anticomplement immunofluorescence (Ito et al., 1976).
Differences between cases and controls have also been observed using
a mixed-hemadsorption assay (Christensen and Espmark, 1976) and by
testing sera against antigens prepared from lysates of virus-
infected cells (Ory et al., 1974), or virus-transformed cells
(Notter and Docherty, 1976). In addition, antibodies to specific
proteins induced by the virus have been quantitated by precipitation
reactions using sera from women with cervical cancer and control
women (Melnick et al., 1976).

While antibodies detected by neutralization appear to be directed
against glycoproteins on the surface of the virus, the exact nature
of the antigens detected by the other techniques have, for the most
part, not been delineated. One antigen studied in some detail has
been AG-4 which has a molecular weight of 161,000 (Aurelian et al.,
1976). The antigen is synthesized early in the replicative cycle
and may be a minor component of the virion. Antibodies to this
antigen were detected by complement fixation in about 85% of sera
from predominantly black women with invasive carcinoma of the cervix
and in very few sera from control women. The presence of antibodies
correlated with the presence of a neoplastic lesion (Aurelian et al.,
1973). Among Japanese women, only 47% of those with cervical cancer
had antibodies to AG-4 as compared to 7% of control women of the
same race (Kawana et al., 1976). A second antigen has been prepared
from membranes of virus-infected cells and called HSV-TAA. This
antigen has a molecular weight of 40,000-60,000 (Hollinshead et al.,
1976) and has been used to detect antibodies by complement fixation
(Hollinshead et al., 1973). Antibodies to HSV-TAA have been found
among patients with squamous cell carcinomas of a number of sites
including the cervix and the antibodies have been detected in sera
of patients with active disease as well as those who have been
successfully treated.

The interrelationship between the antibodies measured by these
techniques is not clear. Antibody titers to AG-4 and HSV-TAA do
not correlate with titers of neutralizing antibodies. The association of antibodies to AG-4 with the presence of a neoplastic lesion
suggest that the antigen may be expressed in the cancer cells.
Since a similar association has not been found for antibodies to
HSV-TAA this antigen would appear to be different. However, Notter
and Docherty (1976b) compared AG-4 and HSV-TAA using the same set of
sera and found antibodies to HSV-TAA and to AG-4 in 82% and 78%,
respectively, of sera from women with cervical cancer. Reactions
were observed in only 13-14% of sera from control subjects. In this
study, antibodies to both antigens were found in sera from patients
with squamous cell carcinomas of sites other than the cervix and in
the small number of treated cases of cervical cancer. Thus, while
non-neutralizing antibodies to HSV-2-induced antigens are found more
frequently and at higher titers among women with cervical cancer than
among women without this cancer, the significance of these observations

in terms of the presence of viral genetic information in the cancer
cells is not yet unequivocally established.

Antibodies to HSV-2 in Relation to Tumor Burden

As mentioned earlier, the presence of antibodies to virus-induced
antigens in sera from women with cancer but not from women without
cancer, the decrease in titer of these antibodies after successful
treatment and the reappearance of antibodies with recurrence of the
cancer strongly suggest that the antigen is associated with the
cancer cells. As indicated, this pattern has been reported for antibodies to AG-4 (Aurelian et al., 1973). Other workers have also
noted fluctuation in antibody titers to HSV-2 in relation to tumor
burden.

It has been noted that titers of HSV-2 antibodies increased with
progression of cervical dysplasia (Sprecher-Goldberger et al., 1973).
A decrease in antibody to HSV-2 was noted among patients with
carcinoma in situ who were successfully treated (Catalano and
Johnson, 1971). Thiry and coworkers (1974) examined sera from
women with progressing or regressing cancerous lesions of the
cervix and found high or increasing neutralizing antibodies to
HSV-2 among patients with progressing lesions. Low or decreasing
antibodies, as measured by lysis of virus-infected cells in the
presence of complement, was observed in these same patients. Thus,
neutralizing antibodies correlated with tumor load and cell surface
antibodies with tumor progression or regression.

Following patients with more advanced cancer than in the above
mentioned studies, Christensen and Espmark (1976, 1977) quantitated
neutralizing antibodies and antibodies to the surface of infected
cells as measured by a mixed hemadsorption assay. In their
patients, low titers of antibody before treatment was associated
with a poor prognosis. Most women who survived initial therapy and
who subsequently developed recurrent lesions which progressed were
also found to have low neutralizing antibodies to the HSV-2. This
was in contrast to recurrences which were regressing in that antibodies to the virus were present. While this study and the others
described provide support for a relation between HSV-2 and the
malignant lesions, the variations in design, methods of assaying
antibodies and results between studies render the data inconclusive.

Immunoglobulin Class of Antibodies to HSV-2

Indirect evidence of continued or repeated antigenic stimulation
may be derived from seroepidemiologic studies directed at
determining the immunoglobulin class of antiviral antibodies. The
synthesis of IgM and IgA antibodies tend to be of limited duration
following exposure to an antigen. The presence of appreciable
amounts of IgM or IgA suggest recent or continuing exposure to the
antigen. Only a few investigators have examined the nature of the
immunoglobulin class of antibodies to HSV-2 among women with
cervical cancer and control women. The results of 3 studies are
summarized in Table 5. Dent and Bienenstock (1974) used formalin
fixed Hep-2 cells which had been infected with HSV-2 as antigen and
indirect immunofluorescences to detect IgG, IgA and IgM antibodies
reacting with the antigen. They found IgG antibodies to HSV-2 in
about 90% and 84% of the cases and controls, respectively. Few

TABLE 5   Occurrence of HSV-2 Antibodies of the IgM
and IgA class among Women with Cervical
Cancer and Controls

| Immunoglobulin | Antigen | Percent with antibodies to HSV-2 | | References |
		Cases	Controls	
IgM	Fixed cells	5.2	3.6	Dent & Bienenstock,
IgA		27.8	3.6	1974
IgM	Fixed cells	28	6	Schneweis et al., 1975
IgM	AG-4	75	–	Aurelian et al., 1976

cases and controls had detectable IgM, however, the difference
between cases and controls in the occurrence of detectable IgA to
HSV-2 was substantial. Schneweis and coworkers (1975) fixed cells
with acetone 4 hours after infection as a source of antigen and
detected IgM antibodies in 28% of sera obtained from cancer cases
and 6% of sera from control. The antibodies to AG-4 were found
to be of the IgM class; the immunoglobulins were separated by
velocity sedimentation and assayed for antibody activity in a
complement fixation test (Aurelian et al., 1976). Again, while the
results of these different studies vary substantially, an increased
occurrence of IgM and IgA antibodies to HSV-2 have been found among
cases when compared to controls.

COMMENTS

Exceptions to the greater occurrence of HSV-2 antibodies among women
with invasive carcinoma of the cervix than among control women have
been reported (Priden and Lilienfeld, 1971; Kawana et al., 1974).
One of these studies was carried out in Israel and control women who
were selected on the basis of having had gynecological diseases had
an unusually high occurrence of HSV-2 antibodies (Adam et al., 1974).
A subsequent study carried out in this population demonstrated an
excess of antibodies to HSV-2 among the cases when compared to
control women (Menczer et al., 1975). Kawana and coworkers (1974)
assayed sera by neutralization kinetics and established a criterion
of positivity on the basis of results obtained from rabbit sera.
They found no difference in the occurrence of HSV-2 antibodies
among Japanese women with cancer and control women by this criterion,
however, the mean K value for the cases was greater than for the
controls. Analysis of sera from the same population by immunofluorescence demonstrated HSV-2 antibodies in 42% of cancer cases
and in only 2% of control women (Ito et al., 1976).

These two instances illustrate possible explanations for the
variability of the results obtained in the seroepidemiological
studies. The selection of the patients to be studied, especially
controls, is an important factor. Another factor is the inability
of the assay methods to accurately detect all past infections by
HSV-2. HSV-1 and HSV-2 share common antigenic determinants and most
studies were carried out using antigen preparations which contained
cross-reacting antigens. Thus, the criteria of positivity for
HSV-2 antibodies have usually been based on relative titers to HSV-1

and HSV-2 antigens (Plummer, 1973). The criteria of positivity were
based upon patterns of antibody observed in immunized animals or in
groups of patients with clinical infections. The validity of the
criteria to detect past asymptomatic infections with HSV-2 has not
been established and the accuracy of the assays may be quite low.

The nature of the antibody response to viral antigens may also
influence the outcome of seroepidemiologic studies. It has been
shown that patients infected with only HSV-1 or HSV-2 develop
antibodies to both the cross-reacting and type-specific antigens
expressed at the surface of infected cells; about 80% of the
activity is directed against shared antigens and 20% against type-
specific antigens (McClung et al., 1976). Patients who have had a
prior infection with HSV-1 and who subsequently become infected with
HSV-2 produce relatively more antibody to the shared antigens while
little or no type 2 specific antibody is produced (Smith et al.,
1972; McClung et al., 1976). Since prior HSV-1 infections modify
the immune response to HSV-2, some patients may not develop a
characteristic HSV-2 antibody pattern. Such patients may not be
detectable by serological means, thus, limiting the possibility
of excluding past HSV-2 infection by analysis of antibody.

Recently, more sensitive methods have been developed for detecting
type-specific antibodies to HSV-2. These are radioimmunoassays
with sufficient sensitivity to detect small amounts of HSV-2
antibody in sera adsorbed with heterologous HSV-1 antigen. In one
report, all patients with past HSV-2 infection were found to have
type 2 specific antibody (Forghani et al., 1977). A second assay
was shown to be superior to the ^{51}Cr release assay but not all
cases of HSV-2 infections were associated with levels of type 2
specific antibodies which could be detected by RIA (Patterson et al.,
1978). The validity of the conclusions reached by using standard
neutralization test was examined by retesting, by RIA, sera initially
found positive in a neutralization test. Of the 19 sera from cancer
patients with HSV-2 antibodies by neutralization, 13 (67%) were
positive by RIA. In contrast, only 4 (21%) of positive sera from
19 control women were positive for type 2 specific antibodies by
RIA (W.R. Patterson, personal communication). These findings
suggest that there were more false-positive determinations among the
controls than among the cases, and that the case-control differences
in antibody to HSV-2 were greater than originally estimated (Kessler
et al., 1974).

An association between HSV-2 antibodies and the presence of carcinoma
in situ or dysplasia has been demonstrated in some studies (Royston
and Aurelian, 1970; Nahmias et al., 1970; Catalano and Johnson, 1971;
Skinner et al., 1971; Adam et al., 1973; Heyerdahl, 1974; Ory et al.,
1975; Pasca et al., 1975; Peltonen, 1975) but not in others (Rawls
et al., 1969; McDonald et al., 1974; Ory et al., 1974). The
variability observed in the results of studies of women with invasive
carcinoma is also observed in the studies of women with preinvasive
lesions of the cervix. Interpretation of these studies is also
limited by the problems in antibody assay. However, taken together
the data from the seroepidemiologic studies support the concept that
infection by HSV-2 is an event in the genesis of squamous cell
carcinoma of the cervix. The application of more precise antibody
assay methods presently being developed to sera from carefully
selected cancer cases and control women should provide a better

appreciation of the significance of the association between HSV-2
and cervical cancer.

REFERENCES

Adam, E., R.H. Kaufman, J.L. Melnick, A.H. Levy., and W.E. Rawls
    (1972). Seroepidemiologic studies of herpesvirus type 2 and
    carcinoma of the cervix. Am. J. Epid. 96. 427-442.
Adam, E., W.E. Rawls., and J.L. Melnick (1974). The association of
    herpesvirus type 2 infection and cervical carcinoma. Prevent
    Med. 3, 122-141.
Adelusi, B., B.O. Osunkoya., and A. Fabiyi (1975). Antibodies to
    herpesvirus type 2 in carcinoma of the cervix in Ibadan,
    Nigeria. Am. J. Obstet. Gynecol. 123, 758-761.
Aurelian, L., H.J. Davis., and C.G. Julian (1973). Herpesvirus
    type-2-induced tumor-specific antigen in cervical carcinoma.
    Am. J. Epid. 98, 1-9.
Aurelian, L., and B.C. Strnad. (1976). Herpesvirus type-2-related
    antigens and their relevance to humoral and cell-mediated
    immunity in patients with cervical cancer. Cancer Res. 36,
    810-820.
Aurelian, L., M.E. Smith., D.H. Cornish (1976). IgM antibody to
    tumor associated antigen (AG-4) induced by herpes simplex
    virus type 2: Its use in location of the antigen in infected
    cells. J. Natl. Cancer. Inst. 56, 417-427.
Catalano, L.W. Jr., and L.H. Johnson (1971). Herpesvirus antibody
    and carcinoma in situ of the cervix. J. Am. Med. Ass. 217,
    447-450.
Christensen, B., and A. Espmark (1976). Long-term follow-up studies
    on herpes simplex antibodies in the course of cervical cancer.
    II Antibodies to surface antigen of herpes simplex virus
    infected cells. Int. J. Cancer. 17, 318-325.
Christensen, B., and A. Espmark (1977). Long-term follow-up studies
    on herpes simplex antibodies in the course of cervical cancer:
    Patterns of neutralizing antibodies. Am. J. Epid. 105,
    296-302.
Dent, P.B., and J. Bienenstock (1974). Absence of IgA antibody to
    herpesvirus in cervicon vaginal secretions of patients with
    carcinoma of the cervix. Clin. Immunol. Immunopathol. 3,
    171-176.
Figueroa, M., and A. Zambrana (1976). El herpes genital en Honduras
    y su relacion con el carcinoma del cervix uterino. Rev. lat-
    Amer. Microbiol. 18, 111-116.
Forghani, B., T. Klassen., and J.R. Baringer (1977). Radioimmuno-
    assay of herpes simplex virus antibody: correlation with
    ganglionic infection. J. Gen. Virol. 36, 371-375.
Freedman, R.S., A.C. Joosting., J.T. Ryan., and S. Nkoni (1974).
    A study of associated factors, including genital herpes, in
    black women with cervical carcinoma in Johannesburg. S. Afr. Med.
    J. 48, 1747-1752.
Heyerdahl, T.D. (1974). Type 1 and type II herpesvirus and abnormal
    cervical cytology. J. Irish Med. Ass. 67, 445-447.
Hollinshead, A.C., O. Lee., P.B. Chretien., J.L. Tarpley., W.E. Rawls.,
    and E. Adam. (1973). Antibodies to herpesvirus nonvirion
    antigens in squamous carcinoma. Science 182, 713-715.

Hollinshead, A.C., P.B. Chretien., O.B. Lee., J.L. Tarpley., S.E.
    Kerney., N.A. Silverman., and J.C. Alexander (1976). In vivo
    and in vitro measurements of the relationship of human squamous
    carcinomas to herpes simplex virus tumor-associated antigens.
    Cancer Res. 36, 821-828.
Honess, R.W., and B. Roizman (1974). Regulation of herpesvirus
    macromolecular synthesis I. Cascade regulation of the synthesis
    of three groups of viral proteins. J. Virol. 14, 8-19.
Ito, H., F. Tsutsui., S. Kurihara., T. Akabayashi., T. Tobe., and
    C. Nishimura (1976). Serum antibodies to herpesvirus early
    antigens in patients with cervical carcinoma determined by
    anticomplement immunofluorescence technique. Int. J. Cancer
    18, 557-563.
Janda, Z., J. Kanka., V. Vonka., and B. Svoboda (1973). A study of
    herpes simplex type 2 antibody status in groups of patients
    with cervical neoplasia in Czechoslovakia. Int. J. Cancer. 12,
    626-630.
Kao, C.L., Y.H. Chen., M.C. Tang., H.K. Wen., and S. Hsia. (1974).
    Association of herpes simplex type 2 virus with cervical
    cancer of the uterus. J. Formosan Med. Ass. 73, 122-127.
Kawana, T., K. Yoshino., and T. Kasamatsu (1974). Estimation of
    specific antibody to type 2 herpes simplex virus among patients
    with carcinoma of the uterine cervix. Gann. 65, 439-445.
Kawana, T., J.D. Cornish., M.F. Smith., and L. Aurelian (1976).
    Frequency of antibody to a virus-induced tumor-associated
    antigen (AG-4) in Japanese sera from patients with cervical
    cancer and controls. Cancer Res. 36, 1910-1914.
Kessler, I.I., Z. Kulcar., W.E. Rawls., S. Smerdel., M. Strnad., and
    A.M. Lilienfeld. (1974). Cervical cancer in Yugoslavia. I.
    Antibodies to genital herpesvirus in cases and controls. J. Natl.
    Cancer Inst. 52, 369-376.
McClung, H., P. Seth., and W.E. Rawls (1976). Quantitation of
    antibodies to herpes simplex virus types 1 and 2 by complement-
    dependent antibody lysis of infected cells. Am. J. Epid. 104,
    181-191.
McDonald, A.D., M.C. Williams., J. Manfreda., and R. West (1974).
    Neutralizing antibodies to herpes virus types 1 and 2 in
    carcinoma of the cervix, carcinoma in situ and cervical
    dysplasia. Am. J. Epid. 100, 130-135.
Melnick, J.L., R.J. Courtney., K.L. Powell., P.A. Schaffer., M.
    Benyish-Melnick., G.R. Dreesman., T. Anzai., and E. Adam. (1976).
    Studies on herpes simplex virus and cancer. Cancer Res. 36,
    845-856.
Melnick, J.L., and E. Adam (1978). Epidemiological approaches to
    determining whether herpesvirus is the etiological agent of
    cervical cancer. Prog. exp. Tumor Res. 21, 49-69.
Menczer, J., S. Leventon-Kriss., M. Modan., G. Oelsner., C.B.
    Gerichter (1975). Antibodies to herpes simplex virus in Jewish
    women with cervical cancer and in healthy Jewish women of
    Israel. J. Natl. Cancer Inst. 55, 3-6.
Munoz, N., G. De-The., N. Aristizabad., C. Yee., A. Rabson., and
    G. Pearson (1975). Antibodies to herpesvirus in patients with
    cervical cancer and controls. In: Oncogenesis and Herpesviruses
    II. G. De-The., M.A. Epstein., and H. Hausen (eds.). Switzerland,
    IARC Scientific Publication No.11 pp.45-51.
Nahmias, A.J., W.E. Josey., Z.M. Naib., C.F. Luce., and B. Guest.
    (1970). Antibodies to herpesvirus hominis types 1 and 2 in
    humans. II. Women with cervical cancer. Am. J. Epid. 91, 547.

Nahmias, A.J., and P. Roizman (1973).   Infection with herpes simplex
    viruses 1 and 2. New Eng. J. Med. 289, 667-674; 719-725;
    781-789.
Notter, M.F.D., and J.J. Docherty (1976).   Reaction of antigens
    isolated from herpes simplex virus - transcormed cells with
    sera of squamous cell carcinoma patients. Cancer Res. 36, 4394-
    4401.
Notter, M.F.D., and J.J. Docherty (1976b).   Comparative diagnostic
    aspects of herpes simplex virus tumor associated antigens.
    J. Natl. Cancer Inst. 57, 483.
Ory, H., B. Conger., R. Richart., and R. Barron (1974).   Relation
    of type 2 herpesvirus antibodies to cervical neoplasia.
    Barbados, West Indies, 1971. Obstet. Gynecol. 43, 901-904.
Ory, H.W., R. Jenkins., J.Y. Byrd., A.J. Nahmias., C.W. Tyler.,
    D.T. Allen., and S.B. Conger (1975).   The epidemiology and
    interrelationship of cervical dysplasia and type 2 herpesvirus
    in a low-income housing project. Am. J. Obstet. Gynecol. 123,
    269-274.
Ozaki, Y., T. Ishiguro., M. Ohashi., I. Sawaragi., and Y. Ito
    (1978). Antibodies to herpesvirus type 1 and type 2 among
    Japanese cervical cancer patients. Gann. 69, 119-122.
Pasca, A.S., L. Kummerländer., B. Pejtsik., K. Poli (1975). Herpes-
    virus antibodies to antigens in patients with cervical anaplasia
    and in controls. J. Natl. Cancer Inst. 55, 775-781.
Patterson, W.R., W.E. Rawls., and K.O. Smith (1978).   Differentiation
    of serum antibodies to herpesvirus types 1 and 2 by radio-
    immunoassay. Proc. Soc. Exp. Biol. Med. 157, 273-277.
Peltonen, R. (1975). Antibodies to herpesvirus hominis types 1
    and 2 among women with neoplastic changes of uterine cervix.
    Acta Obstet. Gynecol. Scand. 54, 369-372.
Plummer, G., and J.G. Masterson (1971).   Herpes simplex virus and
    carcinoma of the cervix. Am. J. Obstet. Gynecol. 3, 81-84.
Plummer, G. (1973). A review of the identification and titration
    of antibodies to herpes simplex viruses type 1 and type 2 in
    human sera. Cancer Res. 33, 1469-1476.
Priden, H., and A.M. Lilienfeld (1971). Carcinoma of the cervix
    in Jewish women in Israel, 1960-1967. An epidemiological
    survey. Israel J. Med. Sci. 7, 1465-1470.
Rapp, F., and C.L. Reed (1977). The viral etiology of cancer:
    A realistic approach. Cancer 40, 419-429.
Rawls, W.E., W.A.F. Tompkins, and J.L. Melnick (1969). The
    association of herpesvirus type 2 and carcinoma of the uterine
    cervix. Am. J. Epid. 89, 547-554.
Rawls, W.E., K. Iwamoto., E. Adam., J.L. Melnick., and G.H. Green
    (1970). Herpesvirus type 2 antibodies and carcinoma of the
    cervix. Lancet 2, 1142.
Rawls, W.E., and E. Adam (1977). Herpes simplex viruses and human
    malignancies. In: Origins of human cancer. H.H. Hiatt.,
    J.D. Watson and J.A. Winsten (eds.). Cold Spring Harbor
    Laboratories pp 1133-1155.
Rawls, W.E., S. Bacchetti., and F.L. Graham (1977). Relation of
    herpes simplex viruses to human malignancies. Current Topics
    in Microbiol. and Immunol. 77, 71-95.
Roizman, B.A., and D. Furlong (1974). The replication of herpes-
    viruses. In: Comprehensive Virology V. 3, Ch. 4. H. Frenkel-
    Conrat and R.R. Wagner, (eds.). Plenum Press, New York, N.Y.
    pp. 229-403.

Royston, I., and L. Aurelian (1970). The association of genital
    herpesvirus with cervical atypia and carcinoma in situ.
    Am. J. Epid. 91, 531-538.
Schneweis, K.E., A. Haag., A. Lehmköster., and V. Kaenig (1975).
    Seroimmunological investigations in patients with cervical
    cancer: higher rates of HSV-2 antibodies than in syphilis
    patients and evidence of IgM antibodies to an early HSV-2
    antigen. In: Oncogenesis and Herpesvirus II. G. DeThe.,
    M. A. Epstein., and H. Hausen (eds.). Switzerland, IARC
    Scientific Publication No. 11 pp. 53-57.
Skinner, G.R.B., M.E. Thouless., and J.A. Jordan (1971). Antibodies
    to type 1 and type 2 herpesvirus in women with abnormal cervical
    cytology. J. Obstet. Gynecol. Brit. Commonwealth 78, 1031-1038.
Smith, J.W., E. Adam., J.L. Melnick., and W.E. Rawls (1972). Use
    of the ^{51}Cr release test to demonstrate patterns of antibody
    response in humans to herpesvirus types 1 and 2. J. Immunol.
    109, 554-564.
Sprecher-Goldberger, S., L. Thiry., J.P. Cattoor., R. Hooghe.,
    and J. Pestcan (1970). Herpesvirus type 2 infection and
    carcinoma of the cervix. Lancet. 2, 266.
Sprecher-Goldberger, S., L. Thiry., I. Gould., Y. Fassin., and
    C. Gompel (1973). Increasing antibody titers to herpes
    simplex virus type 2 during follow-up of women with cervical
    dysplasia. Am. J. Epid. 97, 103-110.
Thiry, L., S. Sprecher-Goldberger., Y. Fassin., I. Gould., C.
    Compel., J. Pestiau., and F. De Halleux (1974). Variations of
    cytotoxic antibodies to cells with herpes simplex antigens in
    women with progressing or regressing cancerous lesions of the
    cervix. Am. J. Epid. 100, 251-261.
Vestergaard, B.F., A. Hornsleth., and S.N. Pedersen (1972).
    Occurrence of herpes and adenovirus antibodies in patients with
    carcinoma of the cervix uteri. Cancer. 30, 68-74.

Seroepidemiology of Hepatitis B Virus
Related Antigens and Alphafetoproteins

Kusuya Nishioka

*Tokyo Metropolitan Institute of Medical Science 3-18, Honkomagome,
Bunkyo-ku, Tokyo 113, Japan*

ABSTRACT

By seroepidemiological studies, close association of hepatocellular carcinoma and
persistent hepatitis B virus infection has been demonstrated. Route of persistent
hepatitis B virus infection and time sequence of hepatitis B virus infection and
development of hepatoma are reviewed.
Key words: Seroepidemiology, Hepatitis B Virus, Persistent Infection,Hepatocellular
Carcinoma, Liver Cirrhosis, Alphafetoprotein

INTRODUCTION

Among biological and chemical agents which may cause chronic active hepatitis and
hepatocellular carcinoma (HCC), the most important and common triggering factor is
infection with hepatitis B virus. No evidence was described with hepatitis A
virus. A possibility of non A non B virus has been postulated but no substantial
proof has been obtained yet.

A sequential progression from chronic active hepatitis, through liver cirrhosis or
directly to HCC has been observed with chronic infection with hepatitis B virus
and recent progress in this field showed a possibility to control these sequential
diseases by intervening the rout of infection of hepatitis B virus. Therefore
among chemical as well as biological agents, the agent most directly associated
with chronic liver diseases and hepatoma having possibility to be controled is
"hepatitis B virus" infection.

Hepatitis B virus (HBV) is a new type DNA virus with 42 nm diameter. HBs antigen
is present on the surface of the virus and HB_c antigen is on the core of the virus.
HBe antigen is in the inner side of core of HBV. DNA is demonstrated to be directly extruded from the core. Since various methods have been applied and developed
for detection of various components of hepatitis B virus, significance of each antigen antibody system has been disclosed. HBs antigen is "alarm for existence of
HB virus", HBs antibody means presence of past HBV infection and protective antibody against HBV infection. By measuring HBc antibody, chronic persistent infection and acute transient infection can be differentiated. HBe antigen is a marker
of high infectivity of the HB virus. Subtypes of HBV, adw, adr, ayw and ayr can
contribute to follow up the route of infection. HBc and DNA polymerase activity
show the presence of HBV directly. Employing these markers, the close association

of HBV infection and HCC has been demonstrated.

RESULTS

Association of HBV Infection and Hepatocellular Carcinoma

Through collaborative studies in Asia, Africa and the Pacific areas where the HCC
is prevalent, an excess prevalence of HBV markers particularly HBs Ag and anti HBc,
has been demonstrated in patients with HCC when compared with matched controls including other cancer patients or the general population upon examination by highly
sensitive techniques, such as immune adherence hemagglutination (IAHA), radio imm-
unoassay or reversed passive hemagglutination. Higher prevalence of persistent
HBs antigenemia and high titer of anti-HBc, over 2^{10} by IAHA, have shown that
larger proportions, ranging from 60 to 90 % of HCC showed evidence of chronic HBV
infection, indicating the history of long-term virus multiplication in patients with
HCC.

Relative risk of HBs Ag positive group to HCC is calculated as 24-80 times
higher as compared to HBs Ag negative group, while relative risk of HBs Ab positive group is as low as 0.3 compared to HBs Ab negative group. Therefore, extremely high risk group to HCC is identified as HBs Ag positive group and low risk group
to HCC is as HBs Ab positive group.

The sum of HBs Ag positive rate and HBs Ab positive rate as determined by highly
sensitive technique will give the exposure rate to HBV among the population. HBs
antigenemia rate is calculated as HBs antigen positive rate among the populations
exposed to HBV. HBs antigenemia rate in HCC patient is 80 - 100 % in different
countries throughout Asia, Africa and the Pacific areas while that in general population is 10-30 %.

The above mentioned data showed close association of persistant HBV infection and
HCC standing on seroepidemiological analysis in HCC prevalent areas.

Relationship between AFP and HBs Antigen in the Sera of Hepatocellular Cancer Patients

The relationship between the prevalence of HBs antigen as detected by IAHA in the
sera of hepatocellular cancer patients and AFP examined. It was found that 74 out
of 169 AFP-positive hepatocellular cancer cases showed the presence of HBs antigen
in sera, considerably higher than the 7 out of 40 cases of AFP-negative hepatocellular cancer, showing significance at the 1% level. Except for 2 transient HBs
positive cases which turned negative 1 month after blood transfusion, sera from
9 infantile hepatocellular cancers and 5 embryonal carcinoma which contained a
large amount of AFP gave negative HBs antigen.

When the amount of HBs antigen was plotted according to the antigen titer determined by IAHA, it was found that adult hepatocellular cancer cases with a larger
amount of AFP, more than 30 ug/ml, were found in cases with less HBs antigen titer
in the sera, showing a peak at 64. Cases with less AFP(less than 30 ug/ml) showed
a distribution pattern with a peak at an HBs antigen titer of 256. As mentioned
above, no persistence of HBs antigen was found in infantile liver cancer and
teratocarcinoma with a large amount of AFP in the sera.

Two Types of HBV Infection

Two types of HBV infection are now classified according to immunochemical flow
analysis of HBs, HBc and HBe antigen antibody system.

The first acute or transient infection is characterized as follows. After primary exposure to HBV in immunologically mature host, transient HBs antigenemia (possibly HBe Ag) is followed by clinical manifestation of hepatitis with a rather long incubation period. Then, anti HBc (possibly anti HBe) and anti HBs antibody response occur resulting in healing of hepatitis, in a similar pattern to infectious mononucleosis with EB virus. The titer of anti HBc usually does not exceed over 2^{10} by IAHA.

The second, chronic infection is characterized by persistent HBs antigenemia, persistent anti HBc with high titer over 2^{10} IAHA unit, and very rare anti HBs response. Clinical symptoms of hepatitis are often observed as exacerbation of chronic HB infection with positive HBe. In such cases, differential diagnosis from the first type, acute hepatitis due to HBV acute infection, is very difficult clinically without measurements of these immunological markers of HBV. Characteristic pattern of these HBV markers in a series of liver diseases, chronic active hepatitis, post-viral hepatitic liver cirrhosis and HCC falls into the second type, i. e. chronic HBV infection.

The second, chronic or persistent type infection which occurs after exposure of the virus to immunologically immature newborn babies or to immunologically incompetent host induced by viral infection such as measles or rubella or other deseases. Most asymptomatic HBV carriers ranging from 3 to 15% of the general population in various countries are due to this type of infection and HCC is closely associated. By serological diagnosis, it is clearly shown that these persistent infections show significantly higher anti HBc titer over 2^{10}, which means long term booster effect of HBc production in the host and can be diffentiated from acute type infection with lower anti HBc titre.

Route of Primary Exposure in Chronic Persistent Infection with HBV

To clarify the route of primary exposure to HBV in the second type, i.e. chronic HBV infection is a very important problem in the control of these chronic liver diseases as well as to control the reservoir of HBV in mankind: over 2 million in our country as well as 120 million in our planet. Three main approaches to this problem have been carried out.

Distribution of HB virus infection classified by subtypes (adw, adr, ayw and ayr) shows characteristic patterns over the world. This was done through WHO collaboration study among Asia, Africa and Pacific areas as well as in Europe and America. adw is predominant in south Asia, such as Sumatra, Java, South China, Taiwan, Okinawa and Amami. Also in East coast Africa, east from Nile River. On the contrary, ayw is demonstrated mainly in Central Africa, West Africa, North Africa, Italy, East Medeterian areas, East Europe including USSR, Israel, Arab, Iran, Pakistan to India. Borderline between India and Burma is borderline of ayw and adw. adr is predominant in Burma, Thailand, Malaysia, Singapore, North China, Korea, Kyushu and Honshu in our country. adr seen in Jakarta is from Chinese. If we further examined subtype distribution of adw and adr in Japan comparing to Korea and China, very characteristic pattern was observed. In Pusan and Seoul, all adr just like in North China. In Iki and Tsushima, they are all adr. In Kyushu, more than 90% adr. In western Japan, adr is much higher than East North Japan and typical North-South gradient of adr was observed in an opposite way to other parts of the world. To explain characteristic pattern, we assume that in Japan, first peoples from South East Asia came through Philippine, Taiwan, Okinawa to Kyushu, Shikoku and Honshu. Then afterwards, peoples from North Asia came through China, Korea and Iki, Tsushima and landed to Kyushu. These are "adr" subtype people and they forced the native ethnic groups up to the North parts of our country. In the village in deepest area in the mountains or isolated

island, we found adw predominantly. The immigrants in Hawaii from Kyushu
are all adr but those from Okinawa are adw. Ainu in Hokkaido is adr but
they are supposed to come from Mongol through north connection. In America, adw
is predominant even in Eskimos, Indians and Indio. There seems to be two alternative theories of their origins. The first is that Mongolians moved across over Aleu-
tian to America. The second is that South people moved óver Pacific Ocean to
America. The adw in Indian and Indio supports the second theory because they are
all adw.

This is very unique and characteristic distribution pattern of the subtype of the
virus and could not be found in any other known viruses such as polio, influenza,
encephalitis and other viruses. How does this type of persistent infection occurs?
The first study to solve this problem came from family tree analysis of liver
disease patients carried out by Dr. Ohbayashi, Tokyo Metropolitan Komagome Hospital. They found several families clustering chronic liver diseases including
HCC and maternal transmission of HB virus occured in these families. When mother
is positive for HBs antigen, 23 out of 26 members are HB virus carriers. On the
contrary, none in paternal side. Actually, maternal transmission from mother to
offspring was confirmed by subtype analysis. All adw or adr transmitted to their
offsprings.

To analyse this problem epidemiolociacally, we examined 17190 cases of pregnant
women in Tokyo and found 380 cases, 2.2% are HBs positive. We followed up 148
pregnant women with HBs positive cases and found 39 cases of their children became HB virus carrier, that is 26.4%. Why some population became HBs positive and
the others remains negative in the children born from HBs antigen positive mothers?
The answer came from examination of HBe antigen of the HB virus carrier mothers.
Twenty two cases of HBe antigen positive mother gave HBs antigen positive children
in 100%. If mothers are anti HBe antibody positive, none of the 21 cases of babies became HBV carrier. Therefore, the presence of HBe in HBV carrier mother
is playing a key role to determine whether their children become HB virus carrier
or not. If we examined HBe antigen positive rate in HB virus carriers, we found
clear age distribution of HBe antigen positivity in Japan.

It is noteworthy that about 25% of HB virus carriers are HBe antigen positive in the
twenty year old and 15% in thirty year old group. That means in Japan, 15% - 25%
of HB virus carriers in reproductive ages are HBe antigen positive and they will
transmit HB virus to their offspring resulting in HB virus carriers in our country.

Time Sequence of HBV Infection and Development of HCC

As mentioned before, high rate of HBs antigenema rate was observed in hepatoma
patients in various parts of Africa and Asia ranging from 80% to 100%. These
data shows very strong correlation of HBs antigenemia or chronic persistent infection of HBV to HCC. To analyse causative relationship of chronic HB virus
infection to develop hepatoma, we started clinical follow up studies of HBs antigen positive group of liver cirrhosis to see whether they develop HCC or not.
One such follow up study will be mentioned briefly. The presence of HBs antigen
is demonstrated very early stage before development of HCC as recognized by
alfa feto protein or angiography. The presence of HBs antigen was demonstrated
by Shikata Orcein staining in biopsy material taken from the liver cirrhosis
patient, before development as well as after development of HCC. Therefore, HBs
antigen in blood and liver cells precedes very earlier than development of HCC.
This was also confirmed by angiography as well as by surgical operation.

From 1974 to 1978, for four years, we are conducting clinical follow up study to see the development of hepatoma from liver cirrhosis patients. Among 115 cases, 7 out of 30 HBs antigen positive cirrhosis developed HCC, that is 23.5%. On the contrary only 5.8% of liver cirrhosis group with HBs antigen negative developed HCC. We classified these liver cirrhosis patients according to their anti HB core antibody titer. If anti HBc antibody is over 1024, 23 to 20% of the patients developed HCC within 4 years despite the presence of HBs antigen in the serum. That means chronic persistent HB virus infection is strongly related to the development of HCC in liver cirrhosis patients. However, when anti HBc titer is below 512, only 5.7% developed hepatoma and this figure does not differ from anti HBc or HBs antigen negative group, that is 4.4%. From these prospectives follow up studies of liver cirrhosis patients to HCC, we are now concluding that chronic persistent infection of HB virus is very closely related to development of HCC. To control and interrupt this type of infection is very important to the prevention of not only chronic Hepatitis B virus infection but also to the control of hepatocellular carcinoma.

REFERENCES

Kojima, M. and others (1977). Correlation between titre of antibody to hepatitis B core antigen and presence of viral antigens in the liver. Gastroenterology, 73, 664-667

Nishioka, K., Levine, A.G. and Simons, M.J. (1975) Hepatitis B antigen, antigen subtypes, and hepatitis B antibody in normal subjects and patients with liver disease. Result of collaborative study. Bull. World Health Organization, 52, 293-300

Nishioka, K. and others (1973) Australia antigen and hepatocellular carcinoma. Gann Monograph Cancer Res., 14, 167-175

Obata, H. and others (1975) Continuous monitoring of HBs Ag and alphafetoprotein in patients with cirrhosis and detection of hepatocellular carcinoma in early stage. Hepatitis Scientific Memoranda, H-881

Ohbayashi, A. Okochi, K. and Mayumi, M. (1972) Familial clustering of asymptomatic carriers of Australia antigen and patients with chronic liver disease or primary liver cancer. Gastroenterology, 62, 618-625

Okada, K. and others (1976) e antigen and anti-e in the serum of asymptomatic carrier mothers as indicators of positive and negative transmission on hepatitis B virus to their infants New Engl. J. Med.,294, 746-749

Tsuda, F., and others (1975) Determination of antibody to hepatitis B core antigen by means of immune adherence hemagglutination. J. Immunol., 115, 834-838

Yamashita, Y., Kurashina, S., Miyakawa, Y. and Mayumi, M. (1975). South-to-North gradient in distribution of the r determinant of hepatitis B surface antigen in Japan. J. Inf. Disease. 131 567-569

Interaction Between Genetic and Environmental Factors in Human Cancer

Interaction Between Genetic and Environmental Factors in Human Cancer

M. J. Simons

*Immuno-Diagnostic Centre, 20 Collins Street, Melbourne, Victoria, Australia,
and Immunology (Pathology) Laboratories, 19 Tanglin Road, Singapore 10,
Republic of Singapore*

ABSTRACT

The strong association between H-2 genes and several malignancies in mice raised the possibility that similar relations may be detected between human cancers and the corresponding genes called HLA. Some associations have been found, in particular with cancer of the nasopharynx in Chinese, and with leukaemias and lymphomas in Caucasians. In view of what are now recognised as deficiencies in the design of previous studies it is encouraging that any associations were found at all. It is now realised to be very important to divide patients with apparently the same disease into subgroups depending on whether they are newly diagnosed or surviving patients. This enables any HLA gene association with susceptibility to develop cancer to be distinguished from an association with prospects of survival.

HLA genes are mainly concerned with the body's immune defence reactions. Immunity may be involved in the development and progress of cancer at many levels such as resistance to microbial infection, responses to cells arising with new foreign markers due to viral infection or chemical irritation, and reactions to tumour cells once the cancer arises. It is therefore likely that HLA-association will exist in every malignancy in which HLA-gene based immunity is involved at any of the several levels of disease development. This generalisation can be expected to apply irrespective of whether the cancer-causing mechanisms involve chemicals, viruses or other factors. It is important to continue the search for HLA patterns in human cancers because HLA typing can be applied to many research and clinical problems including recognising risk factors, testing hypotheses concerning suspected environmental factors, elucidating mechanisms of cancer causation, identifying poor survival risk patients requiring better management, improving disease subclassification, and identifying high risk individuals for earlier diagnosis and treatment.

KEYWORDS

HLA genetics - malignancy - disease associated HLA genes - multiple locus hypothesis.

HLA ANTIGEN PROFILES AND MALIGNANCY

The strong association between H-2 genetic type and several malignancies in mice raised the possibility of similar associations between human malignancies and genes of the corresponding major histocompatibility complex (MHC) known as HLA. It was hoped that HLA studies would help clarify the suspected role of genetic factors in at least some human cancers.   The report by Amiel eleven years ago (Amiel, 1967) of an association between Hodgkin's disease and the 4c antigen supported these hopes.   Subsequent studies of Hodgkin's disease and many other malignancies have provided information that is at best suggestive of a role for HLA genes, but overall have failed to reveal associations of the strength that occurs with non-malignant diseases (see Simons and Amiel, 1977).   The fact that the mouse model systems involved multiple genes, including some which were unrelated to H-2, should have tempered any optimistic expectation of simple, single and strong HLA gene associations.   Detection of malignancy associated genes and estimation of the minimum number in a multigenic process is often difficult enough in inbred mice.   Genetic studies of naturally occurring tumours in outbred humans will obviously be far more complicated.   In relation to the HLA system, the complexity is confounded by the fact that HLA tissue typing is a relatively recent arrival in the field of human genetics.   Development of technical and conceptual aspects of HLA genetics is one of the fastest growing areas of medical science.   However, as a result of having to unravel the genetic complexities of the HLA system as we type, and of having to learn how to interpret the HLA data resulting from studies of patients as we proceed, it has become apparent that many of the studies to date should be regarded only as preliminary observations. This is as true of studies in which positive associations have been claimed as it is of those in which no HLA associations were recognised.   In this paper I do not intend to review who found which antigen in what disease, and whether it was found again when the same person or others repeated the study.   This has been done by myself and Amiel (1977), Dausset (1977), Dausset and Sjevgaard (1977) and Lawler and colleagues (Harris, Lawler and Oliver, 1978) in the last two years.   I do want to:

(1)   Indicate those malignancies in which there are good prospects that HLA associations will be established.

(2)   Take a more detailed look at the situation in nasopharyngeal carcinoma.

(3)   Discuss some thoughts on the significance of HLA associations with malignancies.

(4)   Give some reasons why I think that HLA associations are with immune processes irrespective of the aetiology of malignancy and therefore that HLA associations are likely to exist in every malignancy in which immune responses are involved at some stage during the course of the disease.

(5)   Offer some guidelines for improving the prospect of identifying new associations and,   finally,

(6)   Mention some developments which underlie my optimism that sufficient information is available for this field to start to gain momentum.

First, some information on HLA genetics.

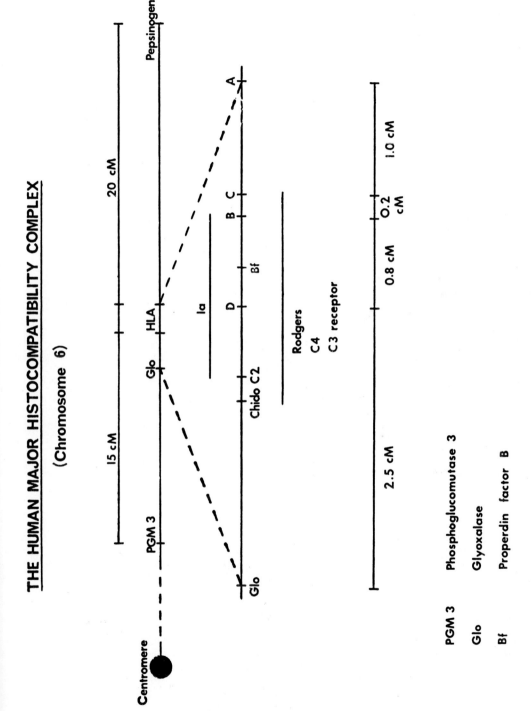

Fig. 1.   Schematic diagram of the major
          histocompatibility complex in humans.

The major histocompatibility complex is located on the short arm of human chromosome 6. This schematic map depicts the 4 major HLA loci which are arranged in the sequence of A, C, B and D since the C locus was discovered after the A and B loci and found to be located between them. Other genes within the MHC region code for complement components (C2 and C4, and properdin factor B of the alternative pathway). Recently, Chido and Rogers blood group antigens were shown to be distinct antigenic components of human complement C4. (O'Neill and colleagues, 1978). Genes controlling the synthesis of two enzymes, glyoxalase (GLO) and PGM3, while not part of the MHC, are in linkage with it. By analogy with the MHC of mice and monkeys, it is likely that genes controlling immune responses exist close to the D locus but the first one awaits discovery.

One of the features of the HLA system is that it is the most polymorphic genetic complex so far discovered in humans. Many alternative forms of the genes, or alleles, have been detected, particularly for the A and B loci, for each of which more than 20 alleles are recognized. Possible combinations of the alleles at these 4 loci number provide for an extreme degree of genetic variability. Caucasians show the most marked degree of heterogeneity. Other ethnic groups show a varying degree of restriction of heterogeneity. For example, A1, A3, A28, B7, B8 and B12 are rarely found in Southern Chinese. The pattern of restricted heterogeneity differs in different ethnic groups, as does the frequency of genes. Some genes appear to be limited to an ethnic group, eg. A1 in Caucasians and the B locus gene Sin 2 (now known as BW46) in Mongoloids.

The term "haplotype" refers to the set of genes on one chromosome. Common haplotypes in Caucasians are A1, B8, A2, B12 and A3, B7. The two commonest haplotypes in Chinese are A2, BW46 and AW19, B17.

Linkage disequilibrium (LD) is the term used to describe an important genetic phenomenon involving co-occurrence of two genes in a frequency greater than expected from the frequency of their separate occurrence. From the frequencies of A2 and BW46 in Chinese, their expected co-occurrence frequency is 30% of 10%, ie. 3% (0.3 x 0.1 = 0.03). The observed frequency of 29% is approximately 10 times greater than the expected. Similarly, the expected frequency of A1, B8 is one-sixth of 12%, ie. 2%, whereas the observed is again approximately tenfold higher. That genes such as A1, B8 and A2, BW46 do remain associated despite the fact that recombination would be expected to bring about their dissociation is undoubtedly a clue to the mechanisms served by cell-surface expressed products of these genes. It is reasonable to assume that linkage disequilibrium exists because the phenomenon confers a selective advantage. Since the major histocompatibility complex is primarily concerned with immunity, the survival value associated with genes showing linkage disequilibrium is probably related to immune responsiveness. Haplotypes showing linkage disequilibrium may reflect the capacity for immune responses that are more effective in terms of nullifying the harmful effects of foreign antigens. Thus, sets of genes showing disequilibrium may be considered as "immune hyperresponder" haplotypes.

Linkage disequilibrium between HLA genes may arise by what is known as the hitchhiker effect in which a single locus situated, in this context, between the A and B loci is subjected to selective pressure, and the effects on surrounding loci are indirect. If this were the case then either the hitchhiker effect is strong enough to bring about linkage between B and D locus genes as well as between A and B, or a second locus between B and D will have to be invoked. It seems more likely that disequilibrium is a result of a direct effect of differential selection pressures on combinations of alleles at multiple HLA loci. This view has very important implications for the ways in which HLA associations with disease are conceptualized, and for the ways in which HLA data in diseases states are analysed. The simplest explanation of HLA associations with particular dis-

orders is that disease associated (DA) genes exist, and that an allele of the DA
locus confers risk for disease susceptibility. It is implicit in this interpretation that risk for a disease will be a function of the presence or absence of a
particular DA locus allele. Consideration of evolutionary aspects of linkage
disequilibrium favours a multiple locus hypothesis with risk for disease development being associated with particular combinations of cell-surface expressed
products of multiple genes, including known HLA loci and genes of loci yet to be
identified. This view does not require the existence of a locus for the development of any particular disease. In 1976 we suggested that "there is no reason to
suppose that the DS (disease susceptibility) 'gene' is coded at one locus. In
view of the existing disequilibria among alleles at loci A, B and D which indicate
the functional importance of a sequence of alleles as a series, one would propose
that the DS gene consists of a sequence of alleles at different loci, preserved in
disequilibrium by their functional advantage as a sequence". (Simons and Day, 1977).
The multiple locus hypothesis envisages that differential selection pressures act
at the level of cell-surface expressed products of the genes. Later the likelihood will be considered that the molecular mosaics of HLA gene products influence,
if not determine, whether any immune response is initiated, and consider some
levels in disease development at which HLA-restriction of immune responsiveness
may operate. The crucial aspect of the multiple locus hypothesis is the requirement for combinations of genes. Thus, the relevance of the multiple locus concept
to HLA data analysis is that the information required is that of HLA gene combinations or haplotypes, and of interaction between genes of different haplotypes,
rather than of the frequency of single genes. Most studies have been of unrelated
patients and have therefore been concerned mainly with frequencies of individual
genes, and occasionally also with estimates of gene co-occurrence, as haplotypes.

There are reports of HLA studies on a diverse range of lymphohaemopoietic
neoplasms, carcinomata and other malignancies. Possibly the best established
associations are those with nasopharyngeal carcinoma (NPC) in Chinese in which the
relative risks are approximately threefold. Hodgkin's disease and acute
lymphocyte leukaemia in Caucasians have also been reported to show associations,
particularly with survival. However, the situation is not clear and the risks
claimed for HLA associations are weak, being of the order of one and a half.
Other malignancies in which HLA associations have been suggested include carcinomas
of the cervix, lung, stomach, oesophagus, breast, liver and melanoma.

Although further investigations are required before the existence of any association with malignancies can be regarded as established, it is encouraging that
any associations have emerged in view of the heterogeneity and relatively small
size of the study groups, the serological problems which have complicated interpretation and the conservative statistical procedures that have been applied in
the determination of significance.

Three general comments can be made concerning the claimed associations; firstly,
the risks associated with the HLA genes are relatively weak; secondly, most of
the genes involved have frequencies from 5-30% among normal individuals; and
thirdly, many of the genes are part of the haplotypes exhibiting linkage disequilibrium in normal populations.

HLA associations in Singapore Chinese patients with nasopharyngeal carcinoma
illustrate these points and hint at the complexity of the situation. When
patient heterogeneity is decreased by subgrouping into those who are newly
diagnosed, and who are younger (<30), and less young (>30) at diagnosis, and
into those who have survived 5 years or more from diagnosis, several associations
become apparent. The haplotype A2, Sin 2 now A2, BW46, only appears to be a
susceptibility risk factor in the patients who are older (>30) at diagnosis
(RR 2.4). Only one patient (5%) of 20 under the age of 30 had both A2 and BW46

in contrast to 40 (33%) of 121 older patients and 41 (17%) of 238 normals. In the
survivors the frequency was no different from normal suggesting that there had
been a relative increase in mortality of patients with this haplotype.

The frequency of the second haplotype (AW19/A.Blank, BW17) which shows linkage
disequilibrium in normal Chinese is also decreased in survivors, suggesting that
it, too, is a risk factor for poor survival. Like A2, BW46 it is also increased
in frequency in patients who are older at diagnosis (RR 2.45). However, it occurs
in relatively greater frequency in the younger patients, being associated with a
relative risk of 6.5. Among the other combinations that have been examined, a
third association emerged, namely that of A2 in the absence of either B locus risk
factors in long-term survivors. Thirty-four (24%) of 141 newly diagnosed patients
had A2 without either BW17 or BW46, whereas 17 (77%) of 22 survivors showed the
HLA pattern.

Associations involving AW19, BW17 and A2 without BW17 or BW46 were only made when
susceptibility for NPC and survival after diagnosis were sharply distinguished as
newly diagnosed patients and long-term survivors. As in studies of acute
lymphocytic leukaemia (Rogentine and colleagues, 1973), previous studies by us in
which we had failed to make this distinction had confounded survival and susceptibility in the association with A2.

The susceptibility and survival risks associated with A2, BW46 and AW19, BW17
seem only to be associated with the co-occurrence of the genes. Risk does not
appear to be increased in patients with BW46 who lack A2, or who have BW17 but
lack AW19. An exception may exist in the newly diagnosed cases under 30 years of
age where the frequency of joint occurrence of A2 and BW46 is lower than in older
groups but where there is a relative excess of BW46 occurring without A2.

Two further observations are relevant to an understanding of the genetic mechanisms.
There is no evidence to date that either homozygosity of BW17 or BW46, or the joint
occurrence of the two B locus alleles further increases the risk. The simplest
interpretation of these observations is that a single dominant DA gene is in
disequilibrium with both BW17 and BW46, and that the occurrence of either haplotype
bearing the DA gene is a sufficient requirement. As described previously (Simons
and colleagues, 1978) this interpretation is consistent with the available data.
If this is a valid model, explanations are required for the observations that the
susceptibility risk of AW19, BW17 is greatest in the younger patients among whom
there is no obvious risk associated with A2, BW46 and, the poor survival risk of
AW19, BW17 is more marked than that of A2, BW46.

Until explanations are forthcoming, the possibility exists that the genetic
significance of each haplotype may differ in the NPC patient subgroups. If so,
it would imply either that there were different DA alleles involved in the two
haplotypes which confer different functional significance, or that additional
genetic loci are involved, the contribution of which varies between the patient
subgroups, or that both situations apply. It will be no surprise if the different
associations of the haplotypes with susceptibility and survival, of A2 alone with
survival, and the possible association of BW46 alone with susceptibility in young
age, are eventually shown to reflect the action of a number of HLA gene combinations.

Based on an analogy with the H2 system in mice and the MHC in primates, it can be
assumed that the main function of HLA-genes is with immune responsiveness.
However, if HLA genes are mainly, if not exclusively, concerned with immunity,
then evidence for HLA associations with disease can be regarded as evidence for
the involvement of immunity. This approach to the significance of HLA associations with malignancy can be summarized as follows:

1. Malignancy is not important to contemporary human evolution since -

    (i)   frequency is low
    (ii)   cancer occurs mainly in the post-reproductive age

2. HLA polymorphism has evolved under selective pressures for more effective immune responsiveness, ie. reflects evolutionary mechanisms.

3. Occurrence of HLA "immune hyperresponder" haplotypes reflects these evolutionary selective pressures.

4. HLA associations in malignancy involve common antigens, especially those in linkage disequilibrium as immune hyperresponder haplotypes.

5. Therefore HLA associations reflect immune processes, irrespective of whether the primary cancer-causing mechanism involves chemical, viral or other factors, ie. HLA associations reflect immunity and immunopathy, not oncogenesis.

It is not possible here to consider the types of HLA-gene involvement with the various modes of recognized immune responses. Briefly, three possible levels of action of HLA-associated immune processes are in the responses to:

1. Microbial antigens at primary infection

2. Neoantigens of infected/chemically irritated cells

3. Tumour associated antigens

Although there is no firm information concerning levels of HLA gene action in human malignancy, the generalisation may be proposed that HLA associations will exist in every malignancy in which HLA-gene based immunity is involved at any of these three (and possibly other) levels. To say again, this generalization can be expected to hold irrespective of whether oncogenesis involves chemical, radiation, viral or other mechanisms.

The challenge is to improve strategies for studying patients with malignant diseases so that HLA associations can be identified. It is clearly important to decrease patient heterogeneity by subgrouping patients according to:

1. Ethnic and subethnic type

2. Time since diagnosis

3. Age at diagnosis

4. Histopathological subtype

5. Evidence of exposure to a suspected environmental agent (eg. EB virus, hepatitis B virus, HSV2)

6. Type of immune response to suspected agent

7. Response to therapy

Prospective studies are preferable since they enable determination not only of whether there is an association between HLA antigens and disease, but also whether any association is with susceptibility and/or survival, and whether there is a relation between HLA type of patients and response to initial therapy.

Concerning statistical analysis, three main approaches for dealing with phenotype data from unrelated individuals and for seeking evidence of HLA associations in patient groups, are:

1. Estimation of individual gene frequencies

2. Detection of alterations in heterogeneity over all the antigens

3. Estimation of haplotype frequencies from phenotype data

Perhaps the surest way of detecting HLA associations with disease is by direct demonstration of haplotype similarity of related (sibling/cousin) pairs of patients (Day and Simons, 1976). Multiple case family studies have several advantages including:

1. Avoidance of the problem of choosing the correct control group since within family segregation provides its own control.

2. Enabling direct estimates to be made of the full relative risk, and the lower limit for the full risk associated with the HLA region.

3. Avoidance of problems where different genes may be related to a disease in different ethnic groups, or where a gene may be related to a disease in one population but not another by considering HLA haplotypes rather than single genes.

There are several developments which improve the prospects for HLA studies in malignancy. These include:

1. Recognition of different types of associations, eg. susceptibility, survival.

2. Recognition of requirement to diminish patient heterogeneity by subgrouping patients according to:

    (i)   age of onset

    (ii)   evidence of exposure to suspected agent, eg. EBV, HBV, HSV2

    (iii)   type of immune response to suspected agent

    (iv)   histopathological type

    (v)   response to therapy, etc.

3. Progressive identification of D locus genes. Ten D locus related specificities are now recognized.

4. Technical possibility of typing A and B locus antigens in serum by lymphocytotoxicity inhibition.

5. Improvements in statistical procedures for identification of alterations in HLA antigen heterogeneity.

Concerning point 4, it is now technically possible to detect HLA A and B locus antigens in 1 microlitre of serum by lymphocytotoxicity inhibition. (Tait and Simons, 1978; Betuel and colleagues, 1978). The immediate practical uses of this facility are in HLA typing deceased patients where sera are available and where access can be gained to sufficient family members for identifying the range of possible A and B locus antigens. Also, where only a single allele is detected, the question of homozygosity of heterozygosity may be able to be resolved. This then enables haplotypes to be assigned directly from HLA phenotyping unrelated individuals.

It is important to try and detect HLA associations with malignancies because HLA typing can then be applied to both research and clinical areas. In research, the existence of HLA associations with a proportion of patients can assist in the recognition of risk factors, can simplify the testing of hypotheses concerning the role of environmental agents in cancer causation, and can contribute to the elucidation of mechanisms of cancer causation by high risk factors. Application of HLA typing to the clinical area can assist in improving management of poor survival risk patients, in better disease classification by identification of different disease subgroups, and in earlier diagnosis and treatment by identification of high cancer risk individuals.

More data from studies which take account of the factors considered in this paper are required before these applications can be more fully exploited.

REFERENCES

Amiel, J.L. (1967). Study of the leucocyte phenotypes in Hodgkin's disease, in Histocompatibility Testing 1967, p.79, Munksgaard, Copenhagen.

Betuel, H., Touraine, J.L., Souillet, G. and Jeune, M. (1978). Absence of cell membrane HLA antigens in an immunodeficient child. Tissue Antigens, 11, 68.

Day, N.E. and Simons, M.J. (1976). Disease susceptibility genes - their identification by multiple case family studies. Tissue Antigens, 8, 109.

Dausset, J. and Sjevgaard, A. (1977). Eds. HLA and Disease, Munksgaard, Copenhagen.

Dausset, J. (1977), HLA and Association with Malignancy : A critical View, in HLA and Malignancy (Eds. Murphy, G.P., Cohen, E., Fitzpatrick, J.E. and Pressman, D.) Alan R. Liss, Inc., New York, pp. 131-144.

Harris, R., Lawler, S.D. and Oliver, R.T.D. (1978). The HLA system in acute leukaemia and Hodgkin's disease, in The HLA System (Ed. Bodmer, W.F.) Brit. Med. Bull., 34, No. 3, pp. 301-304.

Rogentine, G.N., Trapani, R.J., Yankee, R.J. and Menderron, E.S. (1973). HLA antigens and acute lymphocytic leukaemia : The nature of the HLA - A2 association. Tissue Antigens, 3, 470

Simons, M.J. and Amiel, J.L. (1977). HLA and Malignant Diseases, in HLA and Disease (Eds. Dausset, J. and Svejgaard, A.)., Munksgaard, Copenhagen, PP. 212-232.

Simons, M.J. and Day, N.E. (1977), Histocompatibility Leucocyte Antigen Patterns and Nasopharyngeal Carcinoma, In Epidemiology and Cancer Registries in the Pacific Basin, Nat. Cancer Inst. Man., 47, pp. 143 - 146.

Simons, M.J., Chan, S.H., Wee, G.B., Shanmugaratnam, K., Goh, E.H., Ho, J.H.C., Chan, J.C.W., Darmalingam, S., Prasad, U., Betuel, H., Day, N.E. and de Thé, G. (1978). Nasopharyngeal Carcinoma and Histocompatibility Antigens, In Nasopharyngeal Carcinoma : Etiology and Control. (de Thé, G. and Ito, H., Eds.) IARC Scientific Publications, Lyon, France, pp. 271 - 282.

Tait, B.D. and Simons, M.J. (1978). Unpublished observations.

O'Neil, G.J., Soo Yang, Tegoli, J., Berger, R., Dupont, B. (1978). Chido and
    Rodgers Blood groups are distinct antigenic components of human
    complement C4. Nature, 273, 668-670.

Carcinogen Metabolism with Human and Experimental Animal Tissues: Inter-individual and Species Differences

H. Bartsch*, N. Sabadie*, C. Malaveille*, A.-M. Camus* and H. B. Richter-Reichhelm**

*Unit of Chemical Carcinogenesis, International Agency for Research on Cancer, 150 cours Albert Thomas, 69372 Lyon, France
**Abteilung für Experimentelle Pathologie, Medizinische Hochschule Hannover, Karl Wiechert Allee 9, 3000 Hannover, F.R.G.

ABSTRACT

Liver fractions obtained from surgery tissue samples of different human subjects were shown to convert vinyl chloride or related halo-olefins and several N-nitroso derivatives into alkylating and mutagenic intermediates. Although large inter-individual variations were observed, the average activity was in general lower or close to that of mouse or rat liver fractions. However, with N-nitroso-N'-methyl-piperazine, human liver samples were up to 40 times more active than rat liver. When hepatic benzo(a)pyrene (BP)-hydroxylase activity in samples from different human subjects was plotted against the liver microsome-mediated mutagenicity, a statistically significant positive correlation was obtained between the rates of oxidative BP-metabolism and mutagenicity in the presence of N-nitrosomorpholine or vinyl chloride as substrate. Such a correlation may have significance for developing methods to evaluate the drug- and carcinogen-metabolising capacity of different human individuals. Therefore, BP-hydroxylase activity in normal and tumorous lung tissue from 76 patients with lung tumours was measured. A 60-fold inter-individual variation was noted; in most cases the rates of BP-hydroxylation in tumorous lung tissue was lower than in normal tissue of the same patient. When BP-hydroxylase activity in the tumorous tissue (expressed as % activity of the normal tissue of the same patient) was plotted *versus* the number of cigarettes smoked per day prior to surgery, a negative correlation was apparent. These interim results suggest that differences in carcinogenic metabolism may condition in part the response of human individuals when exposed to the same level of environmental carcinogens.

KEY WORDS

Carcinogen metabolism in human tissues, benzo(a)pyrene hydroxylase, mutagenicity, N-nitrosamines, vinyl chloride

INTRODUCTION

With the aim of gaining additional knowledge which may aid in the extrapolation of animal data to man, species differences in pathways or rates of carcinogen

179

metabolism and the magnitude of inter-individual variations in liver and lung
samples from different human subjects were investigated. The enzymic capacity of
animal or human target tissues to convert several carcinogens into electrophiles
was measured *in vitro* using a) tissue-mediated mutagenicity assays with *S. typhimurium* strains and b) determination of specific enzyme activities which are known
to be involved in the activation of certain carcinogens. Comparative metabolic
studies, using animal and human tissues with carcinogens to which man is exposed,
but for which no epidemiological studies or case reports exist, may aid in the
extrapolation of animal data to man. These results may facilitate the selection
of non-toxic drugs (Kapitulnik, Poppers and Conney, 1977) which are metabolized by
the same enzyme system(s) that act on environmental carcinogens to assess in-
directly their *in vivo* rates of metabolism in man.

METHODS

Animal and Human Tissue Preparations

Pooled rat livers were homogenized (3 ml of 0.15% KCl/5 mM Sørensen buffer pH 7.4
per g of wet liver) at 0-4°C and centrifuged at 9000 x g for 30 min. The supernatant was used in subsequent incubations. Human diagnostic specimens with no
pathological lesions were obtained from adult female and male human subjects and
provided by Drs M. Boiocchi, G. Della Porta and U. Veronesi, Istituto Nazionale
per lo Studio e la Cura dei Tumori, Milan, Italy. Human liver samples were prepared within 3 hrs after surgery under conditions identical to those described for
rat tissues. Surgical human lung specimens were obtained from patients with lung
cancer and provided by Prof W. Schindler, Lung Clinic, Hannover, FRG. Normal and
tumorous lung tissues were obtained from the same patient. 12000 x g supernatants
were prepared within 3-4 hrs after surgery under conditions identical to those
described for liver. After freezing in liquid nitrogen, samples were stored at
below -70°C and rapidly thawed immediately before use.

Mutagenicity Assays with *S. typhimurium*

Plate incorporation assay (Method A). Each plate contained 1-2 x 10^8 cells of
S. typhimurium TA1530, 9000 x g supernatant from rat or human liver, an NADPH-
generating system and the *N*-nitroso compound dissolved in 100 μl acetone or DMSO
per plate (Ames, McCann and Yamasaki, 1975). The number of revertant colonies was
determined in triplicate after 48 hrs of incubation.

Assays for volatile compounds (Method B). Mutagenicity assays for vinyl chloride
and other volatile halo-olefins were carried out in assays adapted to test volatile
compounds (Bartsch, Malaveille and Montesano, 1975). Plates containing 1-2 x 10^8
bacteria of TA1530 strain and other ingredients mentioned in method A, were
exposed to a gaseous mixture of vinyl chloride or other halo-olefins in air at
37°C in the dark. The concentration of the halo-olefins in the aqueous phase was
determined by gas liquid chromatography. After exposure, the halo-olefin was
removed and replaced by air. Incubation of the plates was continued for up to
48 hrs and the number of revertants scored.

Determination of Benzo(*a*)pyrene-Hydroxylase

A tissue fraction equivalent to 4-16 mg of wet weight liver or 130-300 mg lung,
an NADPH-generating system and 50 μmol of *Tris*-HCl buffer pH 7.4 was incubated at
37°C for 10 mins (rat liver) or 20 mins (human liver and lung); benzo(*a*)pyrene

(80 µmol) dissolved in 50 µl acetone was added after 1 min of preincubation (final vol 1 ml).   In assays with lung tissue, 1 mg of bovine serum albumine was added. The reaction was stopped and the amount of fluorescent metabolites was determined, using 3-hydroxy-benzo(a)pyrene as standard (Nebert and Gelboin, 1968).   Hepatic activity was expressed as pmols of phenolic metabolites formed per g of wet tissue per min.   The results were calculated from assays performed under conditions of linearity, in respect to time and liver protein concentration.

RESULTS AND DISCUSSION

Carcinogen Metabolism in Human Liver Specimens

The human carcinogen, vinyl chloride (IARC Monographs, 1976) and the animal hepato-carcinogens, N-nitrosomorpholine, N-nitrosopyrrolidine, N-nitrosopiperidine and N-nitroso-N'-methylpiperazine (Druckrey and coworkers, 1967) are converted by rodent and human liver microsomal mono-oxygenases into mutagenic intermediates that bind covalently to DNA (Bartsch, Camus and Malaveille, 1976; Montesano and Bartsch, 1976).   Binding reactions of ultimate carcinogenic metabolites to cellular macro-molecules are controlled by the host's metabolism and appear to be a prerequisite for these compounds to exert their carcinogenic effects (Miller and Miller, 1977). We have examined the nature of the carcinogen-activating enzyme(s) in human liver and the magnitude of inter-individual variations in activities by measuring in parallel benzo(a)pyrene-hydroxylase and microsome-mediated mutagenicity in liver fractions in the presence of vinyl chloride and those cyclic nitrosamines as sub-strates.   Benzo(a)pyrene-hydroxylase activity is considered as a marker enzyme for carcinogen activation which conditions the tumour response to polycylcic aromatic hydrocarbons in mice (Kouri and Nebert, 1977) and possibly to cigarette smoke in humans (Kellerman, 1977).

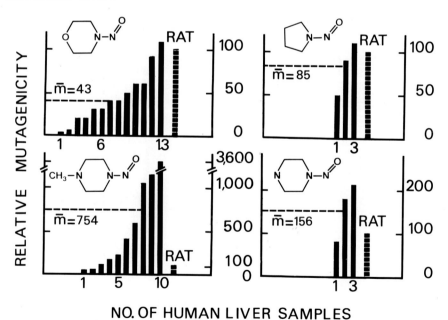

Fig. 1.   Enzymic capacities of individual human liver specimens (solid bars) to convert N-nitrosopyrrolidine, N-nitrosomorpholine, N-nitroso-N'-methylpiperazine and N-nitrosopiperidine into electro-

philes, mutagenic to *S. typhimurium* TA1530. Mutagenic activity
(Method A) is expressed relative to that obtained in assays
using liver fraction from untreated rats (dashed bars) which
is given as 100. Mean activity ($\bar{m}$) of all human samples measured
is listed.

Figure 1 summarizes the relative capacity of human samples to convert some cyclic
nitrosamines into mutagenic intermediates. The results are expressed as percentage
of control; although large inter-individual differences were observed, the average
enzymic capacity to activate 3 nitrosamines ($\bar{m}$) was close to that of rat liver in
which, for example, *N*-nitrosomorpholine is a potent carcinogen. However, with *N*-
nitroso-*N'*-methylpiperazine, human liver samples were up to 36 times more active
than rat liver. If such differences do have relevance *in vivo*, species differences
have to be taken into account when extrapolating carcinogenicity data for certain
compounds from rats to man.

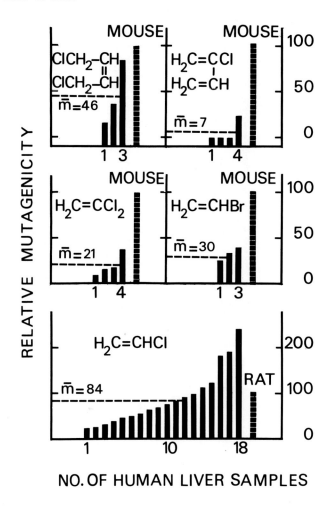

Fig. 2. Enzymic capacities of individual human liver specimens
(solid bars) to convert 1,4-dichlorobutene-2, 2-chlorobutadiene,

vinylidene chloride, vinyl bromide and vinyl chloride into
electrophiles mutagenic to *S. typhimurium* TA1530. Mutagenic
activity was calculated from the linear region of dose- and/or
time-dependent assays and is expressed relative to that obtained
in assays using liver fractions from untreated rats or mice
(dashed bars) which are given as 100. Mean activity (m) of all
human samples measured is listed. Mutagenicity of 1,4-dichloro-
butene-2 was determined according to Method A, whereas other
volatile halo-olefins were assayed by Method B (Material & Methods).

Figure 2 summarizes the relative capacities of human liver samples to convert halo-
olefins into mutagenic intermediates. The results are expressed as a percentage
of an appropriate animal control, which is listed as 100. 18 human liver specimens
were active to convert vinyl chloride into mutagens, the average activity being
close to that of rat liver, where the compound produces tumours. Similarly, human
liver specimens were active in converting vinyl bromide, vinylidene chloride, 2-
chlorobutadiene and 1,4-dichlorobutene-2 into mutagens, the activity being in
general lower than that in mouse liver.

In the present study, we have also compared the rates of benzo(a)pyrene-hydroxyla-
tion with the metabolic activation of some carcinogens into mutagens. Vinyl
chloride, an animal and human carcinogen, is converted by microsomal enzymes into
chloroethylene oxide, a highly electrophilic, mutagenic and carcinogenic agent
(Bartsch and Montesano, 1975) and cyclic nitrosamines are thought to yield alkylating intermediates following oxidative metabolism (Montesano and Bartsch, 1976;
Magee, Montesano and Preussmann, 1976).

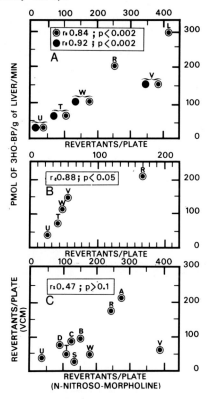

Fig. 3 - a, b, c. Relationship between benzo(a)pyrene hydroxylase
activity and microsome-mediated mutagenicity in human liver specimens

in the presence of *N*-nitrosomorpholine (❸), *N*-nitroso-*N*'-methyl-
piperazine (❶) (Chart A) or vinyl chloride (Chart B). Relationship
between liver microsome-mediated mutagenicity in the presence of
vinyl chloride (ordinate) and *N*-nitrosomorpholine (abscissa)
(Chart C). Tissue samples from different subjects are
represented by different letters. Benzo(*a*)pyrene hydroxylase
hydroxylation was measured as described in Methods. Mutagenicity assays were carried out with *S. typhimurium* TA1530 in the
presence of an *N*-nitrosamine and 150 μl of human liver fraction/
plate (Method A); revertants per 10 μl of *N*-nitroso compound/
plate are plotted. Mutagenicity assays in the presence of vinyl
chloride were performed by exposing the plates containing
S. typhimurium TA1530 and 150 μl of human liver fraction to
the gaseous mixture (Method B).

Benzo(*a*)pyrene hydroxylase activity in human liver was measured and the values
plotted against the respective microsome-mediated mutagenicity in the presence of
N-nitrosomorpholine, *N*-nitroso-*N*'-methylpiperazine (Fig. 3a) or vinyl chloride
(Fig. 3b). A statistically significant positive correlation was obtained between
the rates of benzo(*a*)pyrene hydroxylation and the mutagenicity in the presence of
N-nitrosomorpholine ($r = 0.84$; $p < 0.002$), *N*-nitroso-*N*'-methylpiperazine ($r = 0.92$;
$p < 0.002$) or vinyl chloride ($r = 0.88$; $p < 0.05$). Although limited by the small
number of specimens, the observed positive correlation between the two enzymic
activities would suggest that the substrate pairs are metabolized by a single
enzyme or by enzyme systems which are under a similar regulatory control. Such a
correlation may have significance for developing methods to evaluate the drug- and
carcinogen-metabolizing capacity of different human individuals. Since statistical
significant correlations were obtained between the rates of hydroxylation of benzo-
(*a*)pyrene and those of antipyrine, hexobarbital and zoxazolamine (Kapitulnik,
Poppers and Conney, 1977), such predictor drugs should be explored to see whether
they are useful for assessing the *in vivo* rates of metabolism of environmental
carcinogens in humans.

Benzo(*a*)pyrene Hydroxylase (AHH) Activity in Normal and Tumorous Lung Tissues from Adult Human Patients

Rates of hydroxylation of benzo(*a*)pyrene (BP) were measured in lung tissues obtained
as surgical specimens from 76 patients with lung cancer (study in collaboration
with Prof U. Mohr, School of Medicine, Hannover, Federal Republic of Germany;
Prof W. Schindler, Lung Clinic, Hannover, Federal Republic of Germany and Dr R.
Saracci, IARC, Lyon, France). Human lung 12000 x g supernatants were prepared
within three hrs after surgery under conditions similar to those described for
liver tissues. The patients' smoking habits, drug intake and the tumour histology
are being collected. Normal and tumorous lung tissue from the surgical specimens
from the same patient were assayed for AHH-activity. The results are expressed as
pmols of 3-HO-benzo(*a*)pyrene/mg of protein/hr of incubation. In Fig. 4, the
distribution of AHH-activity in normal and tumorous lung tissues of 76 patients is
plotted. A 60-fold inter-individual variation was observed in the patients, ranging from ≤0.2 to 12 units of AHH-activity. In almost all patients, AHH-activity
in tumorous lung tissue was lower than in normal tissues of the same patient.

Figure 5 shows the relationship between AHH-activity and the number of cigarettes
smoked per day prior to surgery. Very few variations were noted in AHH-activity
of the normal tissue (top). In contrast, when the AHH-activity in tumorous lung
tissue (expressed as % activity of the normal tissue of the same patient) was
plotted *versus* the cigarette consumption, a negative correlation was apparent
($r = -0.15$; $p > 0.1$).

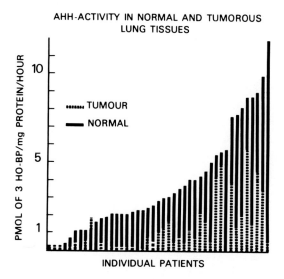

Fig. 4. Benzo(a)pyrene-hydroxylase (AHH) activity in normal and tumorous lung tissues from 76 patients. For more details see text.

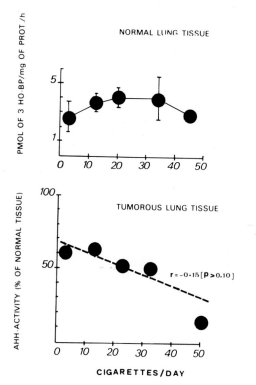

Fig. 5. AHH-activity in normal (top) and tumorous (bottom) lung tissue as a function of the number of cigarettes smoked per day prior to surgery. Results from 76 patients are plotted.

In summary, our results revealed large inter-individual differences in tissue
specific activation of chemical carcinogens (Fig. 1, 2, 3a, b, 4); the capacity
of some samples to efficiently convert diverse chemical structures such as N-
nitrosamines and vinyl chloride to reactive metabolites (Fig. 3c) may suggest that
individuals in the general population exist which are at high risk when exposed to
environmental pollutants; their increased capacity to activate chemical carcinogens
may be environmentally caused or genetically determined (Vessell and Passananti,
1977) Methods for assessing the *in vivo* rates of metabolism of environmental
carcinogens for example by using non-toxic predictor drugs (Kapitulnik, Poppers
and Conney, 1977) should be developed.

ACKNOWLEDGEMENTS

This work was partially supported by the National Cancer Institute of USA, contract
no. ICP-55630.

REFERENCES

Kapitulnik, J., P.J. Poppers and A.H. Conney (1977). Comparative metabolism of
   benzo(å)pyrene and drugs in human liver. Clin. Pharm. Ther., 21, 166-

Ames, B.N., J. McCann and E. Yamasaki (1975). Methods for detecting carcinogens and
   mutagens with the *Salmonella*/mammalian-microsome mutagenicity tests.
   Mutation Res., 31, 347-364.

Bartsch, H., C. Malaveille and R. Montesano (1975). Human, rat and mouse liver
   mediated mutagenicity of vinyl chloride in *S. typhimurium* strains, Int. J.
   Cancer, 15, 429-437.

Nebert, D.W., and H.V. Gelboin (1968). Substrate inducible microsomal aryl hydroxylase in mammalian cell culture. J. Biol. Chem., 243, 6250-6261.

International Agency for Research on Cancer (1976). Monographs on the evaluation
   of the carcinogenic risk of chemicals to man. 11, Lyon.

Druckrey, H.S., R. Preussmann, S. Ivankovic and D. Schmähl (1967). Organotrope
   carcinogene Wirkungen bei 65 verschiedenen N-nitroso-verbindungen an BD-
   Ratten. Z. Krebsforsch., 69, 103-201.

Bartsch, H., A.M. Camus and C. Malaveille (1976). Comparative mutagenicity of N-
   nitrosamines in semi-solid and in a liquid incubation system in the presence
   of rat or human tissue fractions. Mutation Res., 37, 149-162.

Montesano, R. and H. Bartsch (1976). Mutagenic and carcinogenic N-nitroso compounds:
   possible environmental hazards. Mutation Res., 32, 179-228.

Miller, J.A. and E.C. Miller (1977). Ultimate chemical carcinogens as reactive
   mutagenic electrophiles. In H.H. Hiatt, J.D. Watson and J.A. Winston (Eds.),
   Origins of Human Cancer. Cold Spring Harbor Laboratory, pp. 605-627

Kouri, R.E. and D.W. Nebert (1977). Genetic regulation of susceptibility to polycyclic hydrocarbon-induced tumour in the mouse. In H.H. Hiatt, J.D. Watson and
   J.A. Winston (Eds.), Origins of Human Cancer. Cold Spring Harbor Laboratory,
   pp. 811-835

Kellerman, G. (1977). Heriditary factors in human cancer. In H.H. Hiatt, J.D. Watson and J.A. Winston (Eds.), Origins of Human Cancer, Cold Spring Harbor Laboratory pp. 837-845.

Bartsch, H. and R. Montesano (1975). Mutagenic and carcinogenic effects of vinyl chloride. Mutation Res., 32, 93-114.

Magee, P.N., R. Montesano and R. Preussmann (1976). N-nitroso compounds and related carcinogens. In C.E. Searle (Ed.), Chemical Carcinogens, Vol. 173, ACS Monograph Series, Am. Chem. Soc. pp. 491-625

Vessell, E.S. and G.T. Passananti (1977). Genetic and environmental factors affecting host response to drugs and other chemical compounds in our environment. Envir. Hlth. Persp., 20, 159-182

Heredity and Environment in Geographic Variations in Cancer Incidence

K. Shanmugaratnam

Department of Pathology, University of Singapore, Outram Road, Singapore 3

ABSTRACT

Geographic and racial variations in cancer incidence and the patterns of cancer in migrant populations demonstrate the importance of environmental factors in the genesis of most human cancers. Genetic-environmental interactions are involved in most cancers but these are seldom demonstrable in geographic or racial variations in incidence because it is difficult to distinguish the effects of heredity from those of the environment in investigations on large populations living in different geographic areas. The influence of inherited factors has been demonstrated mainly by investigations within specific populations.

INTRODUCTION

This paper examines the respective roles of inherited and environmental factors in the development of cancer from the viewpoint of geographic variations in cancer patterns.

There are marked differences in cancer incidence throughout the world. For cancer as a whole there is approximately a 3-fold difference in risk between countries with the highest and the lowest incidence rates. The differentials are much higher for cancers of specific sites, for some of which more than 100-fold differences in risk exist. If one sharpens either the denominator or the numerator of the incidence equation, e.g. by comparing the incidence levels in specific sub-populations selected on the basis of race, religion, occupation or other cultural characteristics, or by comparing the incidence of specific histologic types of cancers, even greater differences emerge.

These geographic variations have formed the basis of the frequently quoted statements that 75%, 80% or even 90% of human cancers are caused by environmental factors. Although the accuracy of these estimates may be questioned on the grounds that they are based on assumptions that available morbidity data on different populations are comparable and that there are no relevant genetic differences between populations at highest and lowest risks to the cancers in question, these statements have been of practical value in emphasizing the potential of environmental control in the prevention of cancer. Unfortunately, they have sometimes been misunderstood to imply an "either-or" dichotomy between genetic and environmental factors in the etiology of cancer. This was not implied by the epidemiologists who published these estimates (Higginson, 1968, 1975; Oettle, 1964, 1967).

Most scientists would agree that genetic factors have a contributory role in the genesis of most human cancers.

Studies on the geographic patterns of cancer incidence have demonstrated the influence of environmental factors not only by inter-country differences but also by urban-rural and other within-country variations, by identification of high risk groups and their association with various environmental exposures, by the cancer patterns in migrant populations which often resemble those of the countries to which they have gone rather than of those from which they have come, by time trends and in a few instances by time-space clustering, by changes in incidence with age and the shape of the age incidence curves of specific cancers in different populations, by various case-control comparisons demonstrating associations between suspected environmental factors and specific cancers, and in a few instances by the demonstration of a reduction in incidence of the cancers in question following the removal of such factors from the populations at risk.

Geographic variations have been far less successful in demonstrating the role of inherited factors. These have been shown mainly by studies on pedigrees, hereditary syndromes and genetic profiles within rather than between populations. Geographic patterns of cancer may suggest the influence of genetic factors when migrant populations retain the cancer patterns of their countries of origin despite marked alterations in their environment and life styles. It is important to recognise, however, that a cancer risk that is not significantly altered by migration is not necessarily hereditary since migrants often retain some of the life styles of their countries of origin.

GEOGRAPHIC AND RACIAL VARIATIONS: RISK FACTORS

The geographic and racial variations in the incidence of selected cancers and their probable risk factors are summarised in Table 1. The information in this table is derived, for the most part, from morbidity data (Waterhouse and co-workers, 1976), mortality data (Segi and Kurihara, 1972; Segi, Noye and Segi, 1977), studies on migrant populations (Haenszel, 1961; Haenszel and Dawson, 1965; Haenszel and Kurihara, 1968; Kmet, 1970; Staszewski and Haenszel, 1965) and general epidemiologic reviews (Fraumeni, 1973; Higginson, 1968; Muir, 1973).

The observed geographic and racial variations in incidence of cancers of the lip, mouth, oesophagus, colon, rectum, liver, pancreas, larynx, lung, cervix uteri, corpus uteri, ovary, prostate, penis, bladder and thyroid gland may be explained on the basis of environmental influences and are not attributable to inherited factors.

Skin cancer is the best example of the influence of genetic-environmental interaction on cancer incidence. The geographic and racial variations in this tumour accord well with the well known protective influence of inherited melanin pigmentation against skin cancers developing on the exposed portions of the body. Another inherited factor, xeroderma pigmentosum, is responsible for the high frequency of skin cancer among children in Tunisia (Miller, 1977).

Genetic-environmental interactions are probably responsible for the high incidence of nasopharyngeal carcinoma among Chinese and certain South-East Asian populations. The demonstration of significant differences in the HLA antigen profiles of nasopharyngeal cancer patients in selected populations (Simons and co-workers, 1976) supports this hypothesis.

It has been suggested that genetic-environmental interactions may also be responsible for some of the following geographic and racial variations - high risk for stomach cancer among emigrant Japanese (Haenszel and Dawson, 1965; Haenszel and

TABLE 1.   Geographic and Racial Variations in Incidence and
Environmental Risk Factors for Cancers of Selected Sites

Site	High incidence	Low incidence	Environmental risk factors
Mouth (143-145)	India, Sri Lanka, Singapore Indian, Puerto Rico, Brazil	Europe, Japan	Chewing: tobacco, lime, nut, betel Cigarette-smoking, alcohol Vitamin A deficiency
Nasopharynx (147)	Chinese in S. China, Hongkong, Singapore, United States. S.E. Asia - Malays, Indonesians, Dyaks. Tunisia, Algeria, Sudan, Malta	Most countries	? Epstein-Barr virus ? salted fish (nitrosamines)
Oesophagus (150)	Iran, S. Russia, N. China, Rhodesia, Singapore Chinese, Puerto Rico, India (Bombay)	Most of Europe, Israel, Nigeria	Tobacco, alcohol Iron deficiency
Stomach (151)	Japan Brazil, Columbia Singapore Chinese Iceland, Finland, Hawaii Japanese	Nigeria, India (Bombay) U.S. White, Hawaii Chinese, Hawaii Filipino	Salted fish Pickles
Colon (153)	United States, Hawaii Chinese, N.Z. non-Maori	Nigeria, Amer. Indian, Brazil, Columbia, India (Bombay), Japan	High fat/high beef diets ? low fibre diets
Liver (155)	Rhodesia, Mozambique, China, Singapore, Malaysia, Indonesia	Most of Europe, N. and S. America, India (Bombay), Canada	Liver cell ca.: aflatoxin, hepatitis B virus, steroids, alcohol Bile duct ca.: liver flukes Angiosarcoma: thorotrast, vinyl chloride
Gall bladder & bile ducts (156)	Israel, Amer. Indian, Japan, Poland, Hawaii Japanese	Iceland, Rhodesia, Nigeria, Norway, Canada, India (Bombay), Singapore Indian	

- continued -

TABLE 1 (continued)

Site	High incidence	Low incidence	Environmental risk factors
Lung (162)	United Kingdom, Finland, U.S. Black, most of Europe, N.Z. Maori. High female rates in N.Z. Maori, Hongkong Chinese, Singapore Chinese, U.S. Chinese	Nigeria, India, Singapore Indian, Amer. Indian	Tobacco – cigarette-smoking Atmospheric pollution Occupational – nickel, chromium, arsenic, asbestos, coal gas, polycyclic aromatic hydrocarbons, iron oxide ? vitamin A deficiency
Skin (173)	Australia, U.S. White, Canada Children in Tunisia	Japan, India	Solar (U.V.) radiation Ionising radiation Polycyclic aromatic hydrocarbons (soot,tars) Arsenic
Breast (174)	U.S. White, Canada, N.W. Europe	Japan, S.E. Asia Nigeria, Rhodesia	Estrogens High fat diets Radiation
Cervix (180)	U.S. Spanish, Brazil, Columbia, Jamaica, many parts of Asia	Israel, U.S. White, most of Europe	High sexual activity, promiscuity ? herpes simplex type 2 virus
Corpus uteri (182)	U.S. White, most of Europe, Hawaii	Japan, India, S.E. Asia, Brazil, Columbia	Estrogens High fat diets
Ovary (183)	Scandinavia, U.S. White, N.Z. Maori, Israel	Japan, India, Singapore	
Prostate (185)	U.S. Black, U.S. White, Canada, Sweden	Japan, S.E. Asia	
Testis (186)	N. Europe, U.S. White, N.Z. Maori	Rhodesia, Jamaica, Nigeria, U.S. Black, Singapore, Hawaii Filipino, Hawaii Japanese, Japan	
Bladder (188)	Rhodesia, N. America, Egypt	Japan, N.Z. Maori, India	Cigarette-smoking Aromatic amines Phenacitin, Chlornaphazine, Benzidine Coal combustion products Vitamin A deficiency Schistosomiasis

Kurihara, 1968); high frequency of gall bladder and bile duct carcinoma among American Indians (Fraumeni, 1973); low risk for some types of breast cancer,mainly lobular and papillary carcinomas, in Japanese populations (Correa and Johnson, 1978); low frequency of testis cancer in Negroes (Tulinius and co-workers, 1973; Williams, 1975); rarity of Ewing's sarcoma of bone in Negroes (Fraumeni and Glass, 1970; Linden and Dunn, 1970; Miller, 1977; Williams, 1975); high frequency of leukaemia associated with Bloom's syndrome in Jews from Poland and south western Ukraine (Miller, 1977); high frequency of lymphoma and acute lymphatic leukaemia associated with ataxia-telangiectasia among Moroccan Jews in Israel (Miller, 1977); low risk for chronic lymphatic leukaemia in Japanese and Chinese (Finch and co-workers, 1979; Wells and Lau, 1960).

COMMENT

Geographic and racial variations in cancer incidence are primarily due to environmental factors. This conclusion does not preclude a contributory influence of inherited factors. The entry of environmental carcinogens into the body, their elimination, their metabolic activation, their localization in target organs and the development of cancers in specific tissues are, all of them, processes that may be influenced by endogenous host factors. There can be no doubt that at least some of these factors may be inherited. The development of cancer, like that of most diseases, involves close interaction between heredity and environment. It is not possible to refer to one without allowing for the simultaneous operation of the other.

Some of the environmental factors responsible for cancer in man have been identified and the levels of exposure to some of these known carcinogens may be correlated with observed geographic variations in cancer incidence. However, the distribution of cancer among individuals in any given population is not always correlated with the levels of their exposures to such carcinogens. Individual susceptibility and/or individual resistance may not be explained only on the basis of "chance" or of multi-factorial environmental influences. They may also quite reasonably be explained on the basis of genetic differences. Inherited factors may influence the levels of exposure to environmental carcinogens that individuals are able to tolerate before the development of cancer.

Genetic-environmental interactions are involved in most human cancers but they are seldom demonstrable in geographic or racial variations in incidence because it is difficult to distinguish the effects of heredity from those of the environment in investigations on large populations living in different geographic areas. The influence of inherited factors in human cancers has been demonstrated mainly by pedigree studies within specific populations.

REFERENCES

Correa, P., and Johnson, W.D. (1978). International Variation in the Histology of Breast Carcinoma. In P. Correa and W.D. Johnson (Eds.), An International Survey of Distributions of Histologic Types of Breast Cancers. UICC, Geneva. pp. 36-65.

Finch, S.C., Hoshino, T., Itoga, T., Ichimaru, M., and Ingram, R.J. Jr. (1969). Chronic Lymphocytic Leukaemia in Hiroshima and Nagasaki, Japan. Blood, 33, 79-86.

Fraumeni, J.F. Jr. (1973). Genetic Determinants of Cancer. In R. Doll and I. Vodopija (Eds.), Host Environment Interactions in the Etiology of Cancer in Man. IARC, Lyon. pp. 49-55.

Fraumeni, J.F. Jr., and Glass, A.G. (1970). Rarity of Ewing's Sarcoma among U.S. Negro Children. Lancet, 1, 366-367.

Haenszel, W. (1961). Cancer Mortality Among the Foreign-Born in the United States.
    J. natn. Cancer Inst., 26, 37-132.
Haenszel, W., and Dawson, E.A. (1965). A Note on Mortality from Cancer of the
    Colon and Rectum in the United States. Cancer, 18, 265-272.
Haenszel, W., and Kurihara, M. (1968).   Studies of Japanese Migrants. I. Mortality
    from Cancer and Other Diseases Among Japanese in the United States. J. natn.
    Cancer Inst., 40, 43-68.
Higginson, J. (1968). Present Trends in Cancer Epidemiology. In Proceedings of
    8th Canadian Cancer Conference. Honey Harbor, Ontario. pp. 40-75.
Higginson, J. (1975). Cancer Etiology and Prevention. In J.F. Fraumeni Jr. (Ed.),
    Persons at High Risk of Cancer. Academic Press, New York. pp. 385-397.
Kmet, J. (1970). The Role of Migrant Populations in Studies of Selected Cancer
    Sites: A Review. J. chron. Dis., 23, 305-324.
Linden, G., and Dunn, J.E. (1970). Ewing's Sarcoma in Negroes. Lancet, 1, 1171.
Miller, R.W. (1977). Ethnic Differences in Cancer Occurrence: Genetic and
    Environmental Influences with Particular Reference to Neuroblastoma. In J.J.
    Mulvihill, R.W. Miller and J.F. Fraumeni Jr. (Eds.), Genetics of Human Cancer.
    Raven Press, N.Y. pp. 1-14.
Muir, C.S. (1973). Geographical Differences in Cancer Patterns. In R. Doll and
    I. Vodopija (Eds.), Host Environment Interactions in the Etiology of Cancer
    in Man. IARC, Lyon. pp. 1-13.
Oettle, A.G. (1964). Cancer in Africa, especially in Regions South of the Sahara.
    J. natn. Cancer Inst., 33, 383-436.
Oettle, A.G. (1967). Genetics and Cancer. International Pathology. Bull. int.
    Acad. Path., 8, 23-26 & 55-57.
Segi, M., and Kurihara, M. (1972). Cancer Mortality for Selected Sites in 24
    Countries, No. 6 (1966-1967), Japan Cancer Society, Tokyo.
Segi, M., Noye, H., and Segi, R. (1977). Age-Adjusted Death Rates for Cancer for
    Selected Sites (A Classification) in 43 Countries in 1972. Segi Institute of
    Cancer Epidemiology, Nagoya, Japan.
Simons, M.J., Wee, G.B., Goh, E.H., Chan, S.H., Shanmugaratnam, K., Day, N.E., and
    de The, G. (1976). Immunogenetic Aspects of Nasopharyngeal Carcinoma. IV.
    Increased Risk in Chinese of Nasopharyngeal Carcinoma Associated with Chinese-
    Related HLA Profile (A2, Singapore 2). J. natn. Cancer Inst., 57, 977-980.
Staszewski, J., and Haenszel, W. (1965). Cancer Mortality Among the Polish-Born
    in the United States. J. natn. Cancer Inst., 35, 291-297.
Tulinius, H., Day, N.E., and Muir, C. (1973). Rarity of Testis Cancer in Negroes.
    Lancet, 1, 35.
Waterhouse, J., Muir, C., Correa, P., and Powell, J. (1976). Cancer Incidence in
    Five Continents, Vol. III. IARC, Lyon. pp. 453-547.
Wells, R., and Lau, K.S. (1960). Incidence of Leukaemia in Singapore, and Rarity
    of Chronic Lymphocytic Leukaemia in Chinese. Br. med. J., 1, 759-763.
Williams, A.O. (1975). Tumours of Childhood in Ibadan, Nigeria. Cancer, 36,
    370-378.

Genetic Predisposition to Cancer

David E. Anderson

The University of Texas System Cancer Center, M. D. Anderson Hospital and
Tumor Institute, Texas Medical Center, Houston, Texas 77030, U.S.A.

ABSTRACT

Evidence of genetic predisposition has to come from specialized investigations of
biologically meaningful groups within populations. Such investigations have provided ample and convincing evidence of a genetic basis for virtually all of the
major cancer types and sites. However, this should not be construed to mean that
all cancers at a given site or of a given type involve an inherited basis; rather,
such a basis only applies to a certain fraction of patients. The occurrence of
inherited and non-inherited cancers accords with a two-step mutation model, the
first of which may be inherited or spontaneous and the second may be spontaneous
or induced by environmental mutagens. When the first of these mutations is inherited, the number of subsequent mutations necessary for tumor production is thus
reduced and gene carriers are uniquely sensitive to exposure to environmental mutagens. Subsequent tumor development will occur at an earlier than average age and
will also develop at multiple sites. Evidence is thus accumulating pointing to
the importance of an environmental component in the development of cancer in
genetically susceptible individuals.

KEY WORDS

Cancer, genetics, environmental mutagens, mutations, genetic-environmental interaction, dominant inheritance, recessive inheritance.

INTRODUCTION

The current emphasis on environmental factors and their role in human cancer and
the oft-quoted statement to the effect that 80 to 90 percent of all cancers relate
to environmental stimuli has led to the general impression that cancer is primarily
an environmental disease. The results of migrant studies and international comparisons serve to reinforce this impression. Genetic factors would thus appear
to play a minor role. However, population comparisons are generally incapable of
providing evidence of a genetic effect; they involve differences in geography,
cultural and dietary habits, racial and ethnic admixture, exposure to carcinogens
peculiar to a geographic area or life style, availability and use of medical
services, diagnostic capabilities or criteria, methods of recording and reporting
morbidity and mortality data, and others. Furthermore, populations might refer
more to political entities than to unique biological units. Any one or several of
these factors could be confounded with or could completely obscure evidence of a

195

genetic effect, should such an effect be present in a comparison. Genetic evidence has to come from specialized investigations of biologically meaningful groups within populations, where the heterogeneity of patient and tumor material, and the

influence of environmental factors are more controllable than they are in population comparisons.

An impressive number of genetic investigations on cancer have been conducted using either a retrospective statistical approach or the analysis of pedigrees. These investigations have provided ample and convincing evidence of a genetic basis in the origin of the disease. The evidence is too voluminous for detailing here; moreover, the subject has already been discussed in several publications (Woolf, 1955; Anderson, Goodman, and Reed, 1958; Clemmesen, 1965; Knudson, Strong, and Anderson, 1978; Knudson, 1977b; Purtillo, Paquin, and Gindhart, 1978; and the monographs edited by Fraumeni, 1975; Bergsma, 1976; Lynch, 1976; and Mulvihill, Miller, and Fraumeni, 1977). The present report will be concerned with examples from retrospective and pedigree studies as they relate to genetic-environmental interactions.

RETROSPECTIVE STUDIES

Much of the initial genetic evidence came from retrospective studies, wherein the morbidity and/or mortality rates in the relatives of a large series of patients with a given type of cancer were compared with the rates in control relatives or with expected rates derived from population statistics. These studies provided consistent evidence of a two- to three-fold higher cancer rate in the relatives of patients than in controls or the rate experienced by the general population. The increased rates applied to cancer of the stomach, breast, large intestine, uterus, and lung, as well as to childhood brain tumors and sarcomas, and leukemia, but not to cervical cancer; the results for prostatic and esophageal cancer have been equivocal (Anderson, 1975a). The higher rates in the relatives were specific since they referred only to the type of cancer in the patient and not to cancer in general; furthermore, they applied only to relatives and not to the patient's spouses, or spouses and their unrelated controls (Woolf, 1956; Woolf, 1961; Macklin, 1959a; Macklin, 1960).

Risks in the two- to three-fold range have also been considered to have an environmental rather than a genetic basis, particularly since relatives could practice similar cultural or dietary habits and/or share exposure to the same carcinogenic agent(s) (Doll, 1978). But the consistency of the findings, the specificity of the familial effect, the absence of an increased rate in spouses, and the more recent evidence (Anderson, 1975b) that relatives tend to resemble one another in age at onset rather than time of onset argue against the increased rates being the consequence of some type of environmental exposure. A more reasonable explanation for the increased rates is that they provide evidence of a genetic effect. The small magnitude of the effect, however, suggests a multifactorial basis, i.e., multiple genes with small effects interacting with environmental factors having a much larger total effect.

More definitive evidence of a genetic-environmental interaction, using the retrospective approach, was provided by two investigations, one on lung cancer by Tokuhata and Lilienfeld (1963) and the other on breast cancer by Macklin (1959b). Tokuhata and Lilienfeld separated the effects of smoking and familial factors on lung cancer mortality. In a comparison of smokers to nonsmokers, relatives who smoked had a 3.4-fold higher lung cancer mortality rate than nonsmoking relatives, whereas controls who smoked had 5.4-fold higher rate than nonsmoking controls. In a comparison of relatives to controls (the familial or genetic effect), relatives who smoked had a 2.5-fold higher rate than controls who smoked, whereas among nonsmokers, the relatives had a 3.9 fold higher rate than controls. Evidence of a genetic-environmental interaction was shown by the fact that relatives who were smokers exhibited a 14-fold excess of lung cancer mortality than controls who were nonsmokers.

Similar types of comparisons can be made for breast cancer, using the data of Macklin (1959b). She was interested in evaluating the relative effects of genetic and parity differences on breast mortality and morbidity. Previous studies had shown that relatives of breast cancer patients had a two- to three-fold higher risk of the disease than controls, and nulliparous women had approximately a two-fold increased risk compared with parous women. No study had been undertaken to separate the two factors in the same body of data until Macklin's (1959b) study. When her data (her tables 4 and 5) were classified into nulliparous and parous women, the following results emerged: Nulliparous relatives of patients exhibited a 2.2-fold higher risk than parous relatives; and in controls, nulliparous women had a 2.3-fold higher risk than parous women. The genetic effect was also the same whether it applied to nulliparous (3.7-fold increase) or parous women (3.5-fold increase). In her data, therefore, the genetic and parity effects appeared to be independent and multiplicative, since nulliparous relatives had an 8-fold higher risk than parous controls.

PEDIGREE STUDIES

In comparison with the retrospective approach, a much more fruitful method for demonstrating a genetic predisposition involves the analysis of pedigrees. This method is appealing because it provides data amenable to tests of specific genetic hypotheses. Whereas the retrospective approach may only indicate the presence of a genetic component, the pedigree approach does the same but it also provides data on the specific mode of inheritance, variability in clinical expressivity, degree of penetrance, linkage relations with other genetic markers, and it provides data of basic and clinical interest from a more homogeneous group of patients than would be available from retrospective studies. This method has now provided evidence of inherited cancers at virtually all of the major cancer sites (Knudson, Strong, and Anderson, 1973).

Mulvihill (1977) summarized over 200 recessively and dominantly inherited conditions in which cancer was the sole feature, a frequent concomitant, or a rare complication. More recently, Purtillo, Paquin, and Gindhart (1978) referred to 240 inherited neoplastic conditions. In both surveys the majority of conditions were dominantly inherited. Some refer to individual types of cancer that are confined to a single site or cell system, and others to constellations of cancers involving several sites and types. Individually these inherited types are rare, but in the aggregate, they are perhaps more numerous than is generally suspected.

MUTATIONAL MODEL

Knudson (1971) proposed a model to explain the occurrence of dominantly inherited as well as noninherited types of cancers. His model proposes that all cancers derive from a single cell and are the consequence of two mutational events. The first mutational event may be pre-zygotic or post-zygotic, but the second event is always post-zygotic. Either mutational event may occur spontaneously or be induced by environmental mutagens. When the first event is pre-zygotic and occurs in a germinal cell, it may thus be transmitted via the zygote and will be present in every cell of the recipient and will be hereditary. The carrier of this mutant gene may develop no cancers, one, two, or more cancers in accordance with a Poisson distribution. When the first mutation is post-zygotic and occurs in a somatic cell, the mutant will be confined to a single cell (and its derivatives) and will not be hereditary. Since one mutation has already occurred in the heritable type and is present in all cells, only a single second event is necessary for tumor development. The heritable type will thus be early and frequently multiple in occurrence. The non-heritable or somatic type, however, requires two infrequent mutational events in a single cell for cancer development, and as such, it will be later and single in occurrence.

The model has been applied to retinoblastoma, Wilms' tumor, neuroblastoma, and pheochromocytoma, with excellent agreement between the observed and expected numbers of gene carriers with none, one, two, or more tumors (Knudson and Strong, 1972). As expected, the gene carriers had an excess of multiple tumors and an early age at onset compared with patients with the non-heritable forms of the same tumors. The model was also used to estimate the fraction of inherited cancers. Hereditary retinoblastoma was estimated to account for 40 percent of all cases of this tumor. The hereditary fraction in Wilms' tumor was 38 percent and 22 percent in all cases of neuroblastoma.

Adult cancers also appear to fit the model, since they too may occur in a dominantly inherited or in a non-inherited form. Furthermore, the inherited cancers are characterized by a significantly earlier average age at diagnosis and a higher frequency of multiple primary cancers than the non-inherited forms of these cancers (Knudson, Strong, and Anderson, 1973). The fractions of hereditary cases among adult cancers have not as yet been directly estimated. An indirect estimate is available for breast cancer, based on the frequency of bilaterality. The bilaterality rate in unselected patients is about three percent and in familial cases 10 percent. Assuming all bilateral cases to be hereditary, in keeping with childhood cancers, then 30 percent of all breast cancer patients should have an inherited genetic basis for their disease (Knudson, Strong, and Anderson, 1973). For other adult cancers, minimal estimates of the hereditary fractions can be approximated by the frequencies of verified familial cases of a given cancer among all patients with that same cancer. For esophageal cancer this fraction is exceedingly low, for malignant melanoma it is about 5 percent, for stomach cancer about 10 percent, and for colonic cancer it ranges from 15 to 20 percent (Anderson and Strong, 1974). These fractions point to the fact that not all patients with a given cancer will have an inherited basis for their disease and this fraction will generally be smaller than the non-heritable fraction.

Genetic-Environmental Interactions in Dominantly Inherited Cancers

The model proposes that all cancers are the consequence of two mutational events with the first being inherited or occurring spontaneously and the second being spontaneous or induced by environmental mutagens. There is now a growing body of data supporting the model and particularly the involvement of environmental mutagens in the expression of cancer in genetically susceptible individuals.

The nevoid basal cell carcinoma syndrome is comprised of cutaneous lesions and a variety of skeletal defects, all resulting from the pleiotropic effects of a single gene, which is inherited in a dominant manner with high penetrance (Howell and Anderson, 1976). A hallmark of the syndrome is the development of multiple basal cell carcinomas at an early age, averaging about 15 years at onset. As the patient matures the lesions become more numerous particularly on the head and neck areas as well as the trunk and extremities. This lesion distribution is similar to that observed in patients with the ordinary form of basal cell carcinoma (Strong, 1977a,b). This similarity plus the scarcity of basal cell carcinomas in black patients with the syndrome suggests that exposure to sunlight plays a role in this disease. The fact that white patients develop hundreds and even thousands of the basal cell carcinomas further points to an extreme sensitivity of these patients to the effects of sunlight compared with whites in general.

Children with this syndrome also on occasion develop medulloblastoma (Neblett,

Waltz, and Anderson, 1971). The brain tumor is usually treated by surgery followed by radiation. Strong (1977a,b) noted that children treated in this manner
developed an unusual number of basal cell carcinomas in the radiated area, i.e.,
scalp, neck, collar, and vertebral axis; furthermore, the lesions developed within six months to three years after therapy. Importantly, no undue lesion development was observed in the untreated areas of the same patient. The age at which
lesions developed and their confinement to the radiated area were unlike those
ordinarily observed in syndrome patients and were unique only to the treated children. In contrast, survivors of other childhood tumors including some with medulloblastoma but not the syndrome who received a comparable amount of radiation
therapy and were followed for similar periods, rarely developed radiogenic basal
cell carcinomas. The median latent period for radiogenic basal cell carcinomas
in general, is about 21 years (Strong, 1977a,b). It appears, therefore, that
patients who are carriers of the gene for the nevoid basal cell carcinoma syndrome
are highly sensitive not only to the effects of ultraviolet light but to radiation
therapy. The multiplicity of lesions, their short latent period, and their development in exposed areas all support the notion of a genetic-environmental interaction, wherein radiation appears to have led to the induction of subsequent
mutational events thereby leading to the development of basal cell carcinomas in
the exposed areas of genetically susceptible individuals.

A similar interaction appears to apply to retinoblastoma (Strong, 1977a,b). Treatment of this neoplasm involves surgery and/or radiation. Children with bilateral
or the dominantly inherited type of retinoblastoma have a 10 percent risk of developing a subsequent cancer. Many of these subsequent cancers are osteosarcomas
and they develop primarily in the radiated field. These radiation induced osteosarcomas have a short latent period, about 5-6 years after therapy, whereas radiogenic tumors in the survivors of other childhood tumors have a latent period of
15-19 years and are histologically diverse in type. These observations suggest
again that retinoblastoma patients who already carry one mutation are uniquely
sensitive to the effects of radiation therapy, which seems capable of inducing
the second event necessary for cancer development.

Wilms' tumor, another dominantly inherited defect, appears to be similar in this
regard, since patients who received radiation therapy and/or chemotherapy had a
much migher than expected frequency of subsequent cancers, primarily leukemias and
soft-tissue sarcomas (Strong, 1979a).

Osteosarcomas have also been observed at a higher than expected frequency in
patients with Ewing's sarcoma after radiation and chemotherapy (Strong, 1979b).

Genetic-Environmental Interactions in Recessively Inherited Diseases

More long-standing examples of interactions are provided by a group of recessively
inherited diseases in which malignancy is a secondary phenomenon, i.e., the
primary gene defect is responsible for the development of a disease, which pre-
disposes to the subsequent development of malignancy. Two classic examples are
provided by albinism and xeroderma pigmentosum. Affected individuals are pecul-
iarly prone to the development of cutaneous neoplasms after exposure to sunlight.
This agent may also play a role in the development of squamous cell carcinomas
in other genodermatoses such as hyperkeratosis lenticularis perstans, sclero-
tylosis, ectodermal dysplasias, and epidermolysis bullosa dystrophica (Jackson,
Anderson, and Schmike, 1979). Other examples of interactions are provided by the
various inherited immunodeficiency diseases which predispose affected individuals
primarily to lymphoreticular malignancies. These diseases seemingly point to the
production of an immature or defective cell(s), which on continued exposure to
some environmental stimulus or insult may enhance the likelihood of a cell(s)
undergoing malignant transformation; or, the cell(s) may contain intrinsic ab-

normalities, such as chromosome breaks or rearrangements which may predispose to transformation (Kersey and Spector, 1975). A related mechanism may apply to the chromosome breakage syndromes, such as Bloom's syndrome and Fanconi's anemia, which predispose primarily to leukemia (Miller, 1967). A more comprehensive listing and discussion of other examples of genetic-environmental interactions are provided by Strong (1977a,b; 1979a,b), Fraumeni (1977), and Knudson (1977a). Abundant evidence is thus available pointing to the importance of an environmental component in the development of cancer in genetically susceptible individuals.

REFERENCES

Anderson, D. E. (1975a). Familial susceptibility. In J. F. Fraumeni, Jr. (Ed.), Persons at High Risk of Cancer, An Approach to Cancer Etiology and Control, Academic Press, New York. pp. 39-54.

Anderson, D. E. (1975b). Genetics and breast cancer. In H. Stephen Gallager (Ed.), Early Breast Cancer: Detection and Treatment, John Wiley & Sons, Inc., New York, pp. 41-49.

Anderson, D. E., and L. C. Strong (1974). Genetics of gastrointestinal tumors. In Excerpta Medica International Congress Series No. 351, Vol. 3, Cancer epidemiology, environmental factors, Excerpta Medica Amsterdam, pp. 267-271.

Anderson, V. E., H. O. Goodman, and S. Reed (1958). Variables related to human breast cancer. Univ. Minnesota Press, Minneapolis, pp. 172.

Bergsma, D. (Ed.) (1976). Cancer and genetics. Birth defects: Original Article Series, Vol. 12, Alan R. Liss, New York, pp. 202.

Clemmesen, J. (1965). Statistical studies in the aetiology of malignant neoplasms. I. Review and results. Acta Pathol. Microbiol. Scand. Supp., 1974, pp. 1-543.

Doll, R. (1978). An epidemiological perspective of the biology of cancer. Cancer Res., 38, 3573-3583.

Fraumeni, J. F., Jr. (Ed.) (1975). Persons at High Risk of Cancer: An Approach To Cancer Etiology and Control. Academic Press, New York, pp. 544.

Fraumeni, J. F. Jr. (1977). Environmental and genetic determinants of cancer. J. Environ. Pathol. Toxicol., 1, 19-30.

Howell, J. B., and D. E. Anderson (1976). The nevoid basal cell carcinoma syndrome. In R. Andrade, S. L. Gumport, G. L. Popkin and T. D. Rees (Eds.), Cancer of the Skin: Biology-Diagnosis-Management, W. B. Saunders, Pennsylvania, pp. 883-898.

Jackson, L. G., D. E. Anderson, and R. N. Schimke (1979). Genetics and cancer. In L. G. Jackson and N. Schmike (Eds.), Clinical Genetics: A Source Book for Physicians, John Wiley & Sons, Inc., New York (in press).

Kersey, J. H., and B. D. Spector (1975). Immune deficiency diseases. In J. F. Fraumeni, Jr. (Ed.), Persons at High Risk of Cancer: An Approach to Cancer Etiology and Control, Academic Press, New York, pp. 55-67.

Knudson, A. G., Jr. (1971). Mutation and cancer: Statistical study of retinoblastoma. Proc. Natl. Acad. Sci. USA, 68, 820-823.

Knudson, A. G., Jr. (1977a). Genetic and environmental interactions in the origin of human cancer. In J. J. Mulvihill, R. W. Miller and J. F. Fraumeni Jr. (Eds.), Genetics of Human Cancer, Raven Press, New York, pp. 391-399.

Knudson, A. G., Jr. (1977b). Genetics and etiology of human cancer. Adv. Hum. Genet., 8, 1-66.

Knudson, A. G., Jr., and L. C. Strong (1972). Mutation and cancer - Neuroblastoma and pheochromocytoma. Am. J. Hum. Genet., 24, 514-532

Knudson, A. G., Jr., L. C. Strong, and D. E. Anderson (1973). Heredity and cancer in man. Progr. Med. Genet., 9, 113-156.

Lynch, H. T. (Ed.) (1976). Cancer Genetics. Thomas Press, Springfield, Illinois, pp. 639.

Macklin, M. T. (1959a). Comparison of the number of breast cancer deaths observed in relatives of breast-cancer patients, and the number expected on the basis of mortality rates. J. Natl. Cancer Inst., 22, 927-951.

Macklin, M. T. (1959b). Relative status of parity and genetic background in producing human breast cancer. J. Natl. Cancer Inst., 23, 1179-1189.

Macklin, M. T. (1960). Inheritance of cancer of the stomach and large intestine in man. J. Natl. Cancer Inst., 24, 551-571.

Miller, R. W. (1967). Persons at exceptionally high risk of leukemia. Cancer Res., 27, 2420-2423.

Mulvihill, J. J. (1977). Genetic repertory of human neoplasia. In J. J. Mulvihill, R. W. Miller and J. F. Fraumeni Jr. (Eds.), Genetics of Human Cancer, Raven Press, New York, pp. 137-143.

Mulvihill, J. J., R. W. Miller, and J. F. Fraumeni, Jr., (Eds.) (1977). Genetics of Human Cancer. Raven Press, New York, pp. 519.

Neblett, C. R., T. A. Waltz, and D. E. Anderson (1971). Neurological involvement in the nevoid basal cell carcinoma syndrome. J. Neurosurg., 35, 577-584.

Purtillo, D. T., L. Paquin, and T. Gindhart (1978). Genetics of neoplasia: impact of ecogenetics on oncogenesis. Am. J. Pathol., 91, 609-687.

Strong, L. C. (1977a). Genetic and environmental interactions. Cancer, 40, 1861-1866.

Strong, L. C. (1977b). Theories of pathologenesis: mutation and cancer. In J. J. Mulvihill, R. W. Miller and J. F. Fraumeni, Jr. (Eds.), Genetics of Human Cancer. Raven Press, New York, pp. 401-415.

Strong, L. C. (1979a). Genetics in pediatric oncology. Proc. XII International Cancer Congress. Pergamon Press Ltd., Oxford, (in press).

Strong, L. C., J. Herson, B. M. Osborne, and W. W. Sutow (1979b). The risk of subsequent malignant tumors in survivors of Ewing's sarcoma. J. Natl. Cancer Inst., (in press).

Tokuhata, G. K., and A. M. Lilienfeld (1963). Familial aggregation of lung cancer in humans. J. Natl. Cancer Inst., 30, 289-312.

Woolf, C. M. (1955). Investigations on genetic aspects of carcinoma of the stomach and breast. Univ. Calif. Publ. Public Health, 2, 265-350.

Woolf, C. M. (1956). A further study on the familial aspects of carcinoma of the stomach. Am. J. Hum. Genet., 8, 102-109.

Woolf, C. M. (1961). The incidence of cancer in the spouses of stomach cancer patients. Cancer, 14, 199-200.

Present and Future Developments in Environmental Carcinogenesis

John Higginson

Director, International Agency for Research on Cancer,
150 cours Albert Thomas, 69372 Lyon, France

ABSTRACT

The background to recent developments in environmental carcinogenesis
and geographical pathology are summarized as providing an introduction to the requirements of modern societies, including the
important pioneering role played by the Union Internationale Contre
le Cancer in its formative years.

Data from a variety of sources including studies on high risk groups,
geographical variations in incidence, as well as changes in cancer
patterns, especially in migrants, have increasingly confirmed the
important role - whether direct or indirect - played by environmental factors in many human cancers. In certain societies, the
environmental stimuli causing between 30% to 50% of human cancers
have been identified, of which cancers due to the cultural environment form by far the largest group. These include mouth, oesophagus,
lung, liver and skin. The importance of cancers related to occupational and iatrogenic stimuli are discussed not only in terms
of aetiology, but also in relation to conceptual preventative
approaches. The possible role of environmental and other agents in
cancers of unknown origin are reviewed, and the concept of "lifestyle"
discussed.

The implications of recent observations in terms of primary cancer
prevention and future research are examined in relation to the
necessity to distinguish between hazards to which man has already been
exposed, and exposure to new potential hazards. The value of an
approach integrating laboratory and epidemiological techniques is
emphasized, including "metabolic epidemiology" and better extrapolation, both qualitative and quantitative.

INTRODUCTION

Despite the pioneer work of Pott and Ramazini, the possibilities of
primary prevention in cancer control only slowly gained acceptance.
However, in the last 50 years new occupational and cultural hazards
have been identified and controlled, and experimental carcinogenesis
placed on a sound basis. Today, research on the role of exogenous
factors in human cancer is accepted as a major approach to cancer
control and prevention.

It is only right in Buenos Aires to recognize the important work of
Angelo Roffo in environmental cancer research in the 1930s. Roffo's
foresight was remarkable. His wide-ranging research included studies
on tobacco, ultra-violet light, and oxidized fats and steroids, the
importance of which is now fully recognized.

Nonetheless, it is surprising how uncertain scientists were about the
cause of cancer in man even in the late 1940s. Willis (1948), in his
comprehensive monograph, stated that it would be impossible to prove
the carcinogenicity of smoking in man and added that epidemiological
evidence anyway would never convince smokers.

The Role of the UICC

The Union has played a major role in the development of environmental
carcinogenesis. In 1950, a symposium was organized in Oxford,
England (Symposium on Geographical Pathology and Demography of Cancer).
It was attended by many eminent researchers. Progress since 1948 was
outlined at the Symposium, and Doll unequivocally ascribed lung cancer
to cigarette smoking, although not all participants were in accord.

While the importance of the study of populations living under various
environmental conditions was emphasized in providing important clues
to aetiology, one of the most significant outcomes of the meeting was
the concept of the "environment", used in a wide sense to cover diet,
cultural habits, etc., a concept that is only beginning to be
appreciated today under the term "lifestyle".

Within the UICC, a Committee of Geographical Pathology, under Dr
Harold Stewart as Chairman, was created, which launched an intensive
programme of workshops on cancer and the environment. It is
surprising to what extent these workshops accurately forecast many
future developments.

The Committee further constantly emphasized coordination of
geographical pathology and laboratory studies, with a view to understanding carcinogenic mechanisms. The work of this Committee was
most influential in establishing the programme of the International
Agency for Research on Cancer.

I have presented this brief historical review to show that, contrary
to much present day opinion, the role of the environment has not been
neglected by oncologists.

Environmental Carcinogens Today

More is known about the environmental background to human cancer than
is usually recognized, especially in regard to epithelial tumours in
adults.   There is often a failure, however, to distinguish between
cancers for which the environmental background is adequately
established, e.g. cigarette smoking and lung cancer, and those
cancers for which a role of the environment is based only on circumstantial evidence (Higginson and Muir, 1977).   The role of exogenous
factors, however, is much less clearly established for neoplasms of
soft tissue and bone, of the lymphoid and haematopoietic systems,
and of childhood, in some of which viruses are considered possible
agents.

While it was the wide variations in frequencies of cancer in different
populations, and migrant and case-history studies that led myself and
others to conclude that 70% to 90% of cancers were associated with
environmental factors, irrespective of whether the evidence was
definitive or only circumstantial (Higginson, 1969), at no time was
it implied: 1) that the environment was limited to chemical and
industrial carcinogens;   2) that prevention of all cancers was more
than a theoretical concept;   3) that only a single factor was involved
at each site;   or 4) that host factors were not important.

Cancers Due to Identified Aetiological Stimuli

Cultural factors.   The recognition of the overwhelming aetiological
role of certain cultural habits in many cancers has been the most
important development in the prevention of the disease of the last
30 years.   In addition to lung cancer, cigarette smoking has been
implicated in cancers of the mouth, larynx, pharynx, gastric cardia,
oesophagus, bladder and possibly pancreas.   For several sites,
alcoholic beverages also play a synergistic role.   Such beverages are
also directly causally related to cancers of the mouth, larynx,
pharynx, oesophagus and liver.   Tobacco and/or alcohol related
cancers have shown a worldwide increase over the last 20 years.

In India, cancers of the mouth, tongue, pharynx and oesophagus are
related to betel chewing, as was recognized in 1950.

Cancers related to the workplace.   Industrial cancers are important
not only in terms of "point-source" exposures of individual workers
but also in identifying agents that escape into the general environment.   Moreover, the potentiating effects of certain occupational
carcinogens on cigarette smoking may carry a much greater risk than
their carcinogenic action per se, e.g. asbestos.   However, on available evidence the proportion of all cancers due to "point-source"
industrial pollution probably comprises under 5% of all cancers, the
proportion varying according to local industrial conditions.   A recent
report (International Herald Tribune, 1978) ascribes a very high
proportion of all cancers to occupation.   In the absence of further
information, the scientific basis for the report cannot be evaluated.

More recently, it has become recognized that some cancers are "job-associated", being influenced by the social milieu related to the job rather than to direct exposures (Office of Population Censuses and Surveys, 1978). Thus, certain occupations in the United Kingdom show an increase in cancer mortality which cannot easily be ascribed to known industrial exposures, e.g. gastric cancer in coalminers and textile workers, large intestinal cancer in farmers and executives. On the other hand, the increase in cancers of the oesophagus and lung in the food, drink, tobacco and transport industries, as well as in the armed forces, is easier to explain in terms of social environment. In the United Kingdom, when cancer incidence in each occupation was standardized according to social class, and adjustment was made for smoking, or "lifestyle", the differences between occupations were often considerably reduced. Women classified by their husbands' occupations also tended to show the same unusual disease patterns as their husbands, suggesting that factors other than occupation per se are involved. Fox and Adelstein (1978) have calculated that only 12% of the variation in incidence between occupations is due to the occupation and the remaining 88% to "lifestyle".

Drug-related cancers. The problem of medically caused cancers is well recognized, e.g. diethylstilboestrol, chloramphenicol, and will not be further discussed. There is a tendency, however, to consider the role of drugs only in terms of ill effects and to forget both the intended, and possible auxiliary, beneficial effects.

Cancers of Presumed Environmental Origin

In contrast to the above group, the evidence that the environment may play an aetiological role in epithelial tumours of the gastrointestinal and endocrine-dependent systems in man is predominantly circumstantial, being essentially the most valid interpretation of the data (Higginson, 1969). This evidence has been discussed elsewhere, but is based essentially on temporal and geographical variations in cancer incidence and migrant studies (Higginson and Muir, 1977). Although the concept of a multifactorial aetiology is widely accepted, for most cancers in which the causes have been identified, usually a single discrete factor predominates, such as cigarette smoking in lung cancer.

However, for tumours of the endocrine-dependent system, circumstantial evidence suggests that several stimuli are involved, none of which appear individually of overwhelming importance.

Accordingly, two major hypotheses have been put forward regarding cancers of probable environmental origin: 1) that they reflect diffuse exposures to a large number of man-made or industrial carcinogenic pollutants in the environment; 2) that they result from a complex interplay of a number of stimuli, some of which may not be carcinogens per se. It is surprising how many experimentalists still tend to think of the environment only in terms of chemical carcinogens and to neglect other exogenous factors that may influence cancer incidence. That this should be so is somewhat unexpected in view of the considerable research done on two-stage carcinogenesis over the last 40 years, during which the concepts of initiation, promotion, reversibility, co- and syn-carcinogenesis, inhibition, etc., were all developed. This probably partly represents a mental block in transferring results from one line of research to another.

Carcinogens and Carcinogenic Risk Factors

While the nature of a carcinogen in terms of a definitive chemical is
understood, it is often forgotten that there are a number of factors
which are associated with an increased risk of cancer but which can
by no means be described as carcinogens, such as "age at first
pregnancy", "lack of dietary fibre", etc. These today are defined
as "carcinogenic risk factors" and are of importance in considering
the role of lifestyle in human cancer.

General Environmental Pollution

The role of generalized chemical pollution of industrial origin as a
cause of the majority of cancers in modern societies requires
critical examination. Apart from clearly defined "point-source"
exposures, e.g. mesothelioma in the region of asbestos factories,
associations with industrialization are inconsistent and poorly
defined. Thus, in a number of areas, there is no clear-cut correlation between cancer incidence and level of industrialization. This
is particularly well illustrated by prostatic cancer (Higginson,
1978). Apart from the increase in cigarette related cancer and the
fall in gastric cancers, the overall patterns of cancer observed
today in most industrialized and non-industrialized states are very
similar to those at the turn of the century. Thus, the agents
causing cancers today have been present for many years. The fall in
stomach cancer or slight rise in large intestinal cancer cannot
simply and uncritically be ascribed to food additives. Liver cancer
in most industrialized states would appear due to alcohol and not to
industrial agents.

While certain cancers are relatively rare in some developing countries,
e.g. breast, colon and corpus uteri, tumours of the liver, prostate
and cervix may be more common. The demonstration of the importance
of the social milieu in occupational cancers and the lower cancer
rates in Mormons and Seventh Day Adventists involve not only tobacco
and alcohol related, but also non-tobacco and non-alcohol related
tumours. This suggests the role of other factors besides generalized
environmental pollution (Lyon, 1976; Phillips, 1975).

In conclusion, variations in the incidence of most cancers, with
certain obvious exceptions, e.g. mesothelioma, cannot be explained
on "point-source" or ambient general environmental pollution. This
lack of a consistent pattern would suggest that other factors must
be taken into consideration.

Role of Lifestyle

Lifestyle is an ill-defined concept that implies the total interplay
of all exogenous and endogenous stimuli that may modify cancer
patterns, including diet, cultural and social habits, working
conditions, etc. Oettlé and myself (1960), while agreeing that the
different cancer patterns between Africa and Europe could not be
explained by current theory and that comparisons of lifestyles were
necessary to provide clues, concluded that in the absence of testable
hypotheses, the task of describing lifestyle accurately was impossibly
great. This situation is only now beginning to change as new
hypotheses have been developed and certain of the practical and

logistic problems defined.

Diet.   While many equate lifestyle with diet, it is probable that it
only represents one of the factors involved, at least in relation
to tumours of the endocrine-dependent organs (Symposium on Nutrition
in the Causation of Cancer, 1975).   Diet, however, does illustrate
the many variables that enter into definition of lifestyle, and the
mechanisms whereby it may affect cancer patterns :
1) the presence of direct or indirect carcinogens in the diet;
2) an enhancing role for the delivery of carcinogens, e.g. alcoholic
beverages;   3) that diet may be involved in metabolic activation or
inactivation of carcinogens;   4) that endogenous carcinogen formation
may occur from dietary substrates, e.g. nitrates, nitrites and
amines;   5) that diet may affect host susceptibility either non-
specifically due to variations in individual metabolism or through
the presence of biologically active non-nutrients.

Cultural environment.   There is considerable evidence that tumours
of the endocrine-dependent organs are associated with such factors as
age at first marriage, age at first intercourse, menarche, height,
etc.   These factors are often not considered as environmental.   In
fact, they represent the external cultural milieu and thus may be
regarded as "carcinogenic risk factors".   Hopefully, it may be
possible eventually to express these various risks in more objective
terms which may reflect host endocrine status, etc.   Studies along
these lines are only beginning (metabolic epidemiology), but it is
clear that lifestyle has both a cultural and a dietary component and
that the two are closely related.   However, their complex interplay
is far from understood.   For example, while cultural habits are
insufficient to explain all geographical and temporal variations in
breast cancer, much of the variations in carcinoma of the cervix and
ovary can be related to changes in sexual habits.

Primary Cancer of the Liver

The high frequency of liver cancer in North America and Europe due to
alcoholic beverages is well known.

In contrast, in Africa and Asia evidence suggests a possible causal
role of a mycotoxin (aflatoxin) produced by fungal contamination of
foodstuffs (Linsell and Peers, 1977).   Recently, however, definitive
objective evidence for an association between hepatitis B virus and
liver cancer has been demonstrated, and the hypothesis of the virus
as a co-factor is again being seriously considered (Larouzé and co-
workers, 1977).   The point to be emphasized is that these recent
developments required adequate technology to measure dietary
aflatoxin and identify infection by the hepatitis virus.

Cancers of the Large Intestine and Rectum

Cancers of the colon and rectum have been related to beer drinking,
dietary fibre and fat.   The latter cannot be described as carcinogens
but rather as "carcinogenic risk factors".   Their role is not clear,
i.e. whether they increase the formation of intraluminal carcinogens,
promote premalignant lesions, or are markers for more fundamental
mechanisms.   However, there is no evidence that control of these
factors will reduce the incidence of these cancers.

Prostate Cancer

While the prevalence of latent carcinoma shows some correlation with
invasive carcinoma, the differences are insufficient to explain the
wide geographical variations in distribution of this latter. It would
appear therefore that invasive prostatic cancer is largely dependent
on promoting factors.

Implications for Cancer Control

In Figures 1 and 2, the major factors contributing to cancer causation
are summarized for the Birmingham region of the United Kingdom. These
estimates appear to be the best interpretation of the available
scientific data from that country. These histograms emphasize the
importance of lifestyle, especially in women. They also show why the
concept of cancers being attributed to the environment is so often
misunderstood by both the public and scientists, with detrimental
effects on preventive strategy. However, they have been challenged
in as far as the United States is concerned (International Herald
Tribune, 1978). There it is stated that "up to" 20% to 40% of all
cancers may be due to occupation. This estimate is predominantly
based on the very great load of additional cancers it is claimed will
be caused in the future by asbestos and other industrial exposures in
that country. However, if the report can be substantiated by data,
it would indicate that the American workplace is and will be the most
dangerous in the world. Discussion with colleagues in other countries
suggests that the United States estimates are not applicable elsewhere.
Contrary to the claim made by the report, the multiplicity of factors
involved in human carcinogenesis has been long recognized (Higginson,
1969).

I would, however, like to make one very serious criticism of emphasis
and misinterpretation in the report, notably that members of the
public, not understanding the term "attributable risk" will assume
that a large proportion of lung cancers in the United States previously
ascribed to cigarette smoking is rather due to occupation and will
conclude accordingly that this cancer can largely be eliminated only
by control of the latter. I am certain that this emphasis will in the
long term be detrimental to the best interests of cancer control, and
I suspect it has been received with enthusiasm by the tobacco industry
and caused gloom within the American Cancer Society, the UICC and
other anti-cancer organizations.

The report from the United States will of course be evaluated when it
has been published in the scientific literature, but as reported the
arguments used are identical to those used in the past to show that
lung cancer was due to air pollution and NOT to cigarettes.

There are other reasons to control environmental hazards besides
carcinogenesis. Although carcinogenic hazards may have the greatest
public impact, they should not be unnecessarily over-emphasized.
Nonetheless, it is disturbing to note that, despite the increase in
knowledge of potential control methods, at no time have cancer
research workers been under greater attack for lack of success; it
is true that proposals based on sound scientific observations are
available which, if implemented, could prevent up to 50% of cancers
in males in certain societies.

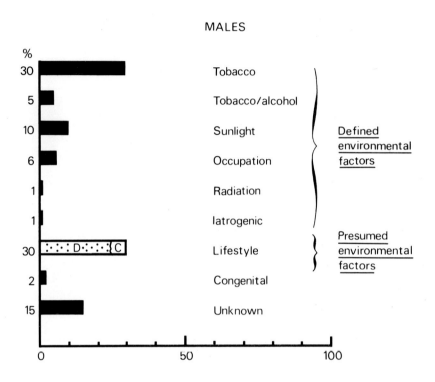

Fig. 1. Estimated proportion of all cancers caused by different
factors in Males in the Birmingham region, U.K.

Lifestyle has been divided into cultural (C) and dietary (D) factors
but no attempt has been made to evaluate accurately the proportion
due to each.

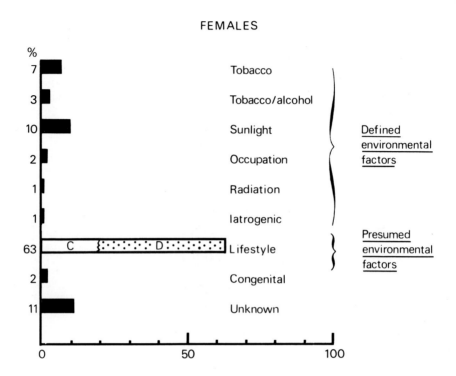

Fig. 2. Estimated proportion of all cancers caused by different
factors in Females in the Birmingham region, U.K.

Lifestyle has been divided into cultural (C) and dietary (D) factors
but no attempt has been made to evaluate accurately the proportion
due to each.

However, for those cancers whose environmental component is only
suspected, or which are due to lifestyle, the data are in general
too circumstantial to permit definitive and meaningful proposals for
prevention. Hence, attempts to legislate or encourage significant
lifestyle changes may prove ineffectual. Thus, those factors that
protect against cervical cancer appear to favour breast cancer.

CONCLUSION

Past failure to control tumours of defined aetiology is due to both
scientific and non-scientific factors. These include:

1) an unwillingness to accept that cigarette smoking is the major
causal factor so far identified in human cancer; it is surprising
that this needs reiteration but the recent report from the National
Cancer Institute claims that a large fraction of cancers previously
ascribed to smoking is due to occupation;

2) belief in the predominant role of industrial pollution in cancer
causation - whether "point-source" or ambient. These exposures are
assumed to be controllable.

Presentation of Risks and the Concept of Safety

The word 'safe' is a statistical concept, and does not mean absence
of risk. An over-simplistic approach to defining risks is dangerous
since it prevents reasoned discussion of the options open to society
in evaluating cost-benefits. Thus, a belief that everything is
dangerous inhibits action against some important and obvious hazards
on the one hand, or leads to unnecessary banning of useful drugs or
pesticides on the other.

The failure by the public to appreciate the scientific difficulties
of extrapolating from animal experimentation to man is responsible
for much of the confrontation that surrounds regulatory control of
environmental hazards. In relation to future putative hazards,
animal studies would appear a reasonable and effective method of
preventing the introduction of potentially hazardous new compounds
into the environment without good cause. The existence of non-effect
levels has been discussed extensively from both a statistical and a
biological viewpoint. There would appear to be supportive laboratory
evidence.

In conclusion, great progress has been made in the past 30 years in
the field of environmental carcinogenesis. This has led to clear
guidelines for both future research and community action. Moreover,
even if difficult, we have at our disposal the possibility of
reducing the frequency of many cancers. However, the latter is the
task of politicians, public health officials and regulators. It is
time oncologists indicated to society and its leaders their responsi-
bilities, as distinct from those of the scientist and expert, in
promulgating and utilizing the available data.

Lastly, we must be prepared to accept that it will be many years
before full cancer prevention will be possible, if ever, and that
identification of lifestyle factors and their role in cancer
causation may not lead to easy solutions.

Fox, A.J. and A.M. Adelstein (1978). Occupational mortality: work
    or way of life? J. Epidem. Community Health., 32, 73-78.
Higginson, J. (1969). Present trends in cancer epidemiology. In
    J.F. Morgan (Ed.), Proceedings of the Eighth Canadian Cancer
    Conference, Honey Harbour, Ontario, 1968, Pergamon Press,
    Toronto. pp. 40-75.
Higginson, J. (1978). Perspectives and future developments in
    research on environmental carcinogenesis. In A. Clark Griffin
    and C.R. Shaw (Eds.), Carcinogens: Identification and Mechanisms
    of Action, Raven Press, New York. pp. 187-208.
Higginson, J. and C.S. Muir (1977). Détermination de l'importance
    des facteurs environnementaux dans le cancer humain: Rôle de
    l'épidémiologie. Bull. Cancer (Paris), 64, 365-384.
Higginson, J. and A.G. Oettlé (1960). The incidence of cancer of
    the Bantu and Cape Colored population of Johannesburg, South
    Africa. J. Natl. Cancer Inst., 24, 589-671.
International Herald Tribune (1978). Study says 20% of cancer will
    be related to work. 13 September, p. 4.
Larouzé, B. and co-workers (1977). Forecasting the development of
    primary hepatocellular carcinoma by the use of risk factors:
    Studies in West Africa. J. Natl. Cancer Inst., 58, 1557-1561.
Linsell, C.A. and F.G. Peers (1977). Aflatoxin and liver cell cancer.
    Trans. R. Soc. Trop. Med. Hyg., 71, 471-473
Lyon, J.L. and co-workers (1976). Cancer incidence in Mormons and
    non-Mormons in Utah, 1966-1970. New Engl. J. Med., 294,
    129-133.
Office of Population Censuses and Surveys (1978). Occupational
    Mortality: England and Wales 1970-1972 (decennial supplement).
    Her Majesty's Stationery Office, London, England
Symposium on Geographical Pathology and Demography of Cancer, Oxford,
    England (1950). J. Clemmesen (Ed.), Council for International
    Organizations of Medical Sciences.
Symposium on Nutrition in the Causation of Cancer (1975). Cancer
    Res., 35, 3231-3550.
Phillips, R.L. (1975). Role of lifestyle and dietary habits in
    risk of cancer among Seventh Day Adventists. Cancer Res.,
    35, 3513-3522.
Willis, R.A. (1948). Pathology of tumours. Butterworth & Co. Ltd.,
    London.

On-going Research and Needs in Cancer Epidemiology — a World-wide Survey

C. S. Muir*, C. O. Köhler**, K. Schlaefer** and G. Wagner**

*International Agency for Research on Cancer, 150 cours Albert Thomas,
69372 Lyon, France
**Deutsches Krebsforschungszentrum, Im Neuenheimer Feld, 280,
D6900 Heidelberg, F.R.G.

ABSTRACT

The 908 epidemiological studies undertaken in 70 countries and reported in 1977 to the Clearing-House of On-going Research in Cancer
Epidemiology, operated jointly by the International Agency for Research on Cancer and the Deutsches Krebsforschungszentrum, have
been analysed. Descriptive epidemiology is undertaken in a fairly
wide range of countries. Analytical studies are much more frequent
in North America, the nordic countries and in the United Kingdom
where there are a considerable number of investigations under way in
industrial and non-industrial high-risk groups as well as case-
control studies. Studies on breast and respiratory tract cancer are
frequent but common sites like pancreas, malignant melanoma and prostate are currently largely ignored. The investment in epidemiological effort is trivial in relation to study opportunities and needs.
The major impediments to epidemiological cancer research comprise :
1) an absence of trained investigators due to failure to teach
chronic disease epidemiology at graduate and undergraduate level,
and to create a career structure; 2) differing concepts of epidemiology; 3) secrecy of death certificates in certain countries, and
other barriers preventing linkage of exposed persons and their
subsequent disease experience.

Keywords : Cancer, Confidentiality, Epidemiology,
Geographical Distribution, Manpower,
On-going Research, Record Linkage

INTRODUCTION

The concept of a Clearing-House of On-going Research in Cancer Epidemiology (CH) arose, as so often happens in science, in several
centres at much the same time. Dr Marvin Schneiderman, the Associate Scientific Director for Field Studies and Statistics of the
National Cancer Institute (NCI) of the United States expressed this
in : "How can I find out what is going on before it has happened ?"
The International Agency for Research on Cancer (IARC) which has the

same need for information of this kind, decided to create a Clearing
House for On-going Research in Cancer Epidemiology. Realizing that
such a venture would require the collaboration of a group experienced
in handling literature abstracts on a computerized basis and in providing information on request from the resulting data base, the
Agency approached the German Cancer Research Centre (Deutsches
Krebsforschungszentrum, or DKFZ) Heidelberg, which has acquired considerable expertise in this area.

About the same time the International Cancer Research Data Bank
(ICRDB) Program of the NCI became operational. The then Program
Director, Dr G.T. O'Conor, evinced considerable interest in the proposed CH and promised support. A mailing list of persons working in
the field of cancer epidemiology was built up and these individuals
were asked (in English, French, German, Italian, Russian and Spanish)
to send the CH a brief abstract describing their on-going epidemiological studies. As the CH has become better known the number of
persons contributing has increased by around 20% each year   (Muir &
Wagner, 1976, 1977, 1978). To avoid loss of information there is a
free exchange of material between CH and the other Clearing Houses
associated with the ICRDB program, viz. the Current Cancer Research
Project Analysis Centre (CCRESPAC) and the UICC Clearing House for
Controlled Therapeutic Trials and material included in the CH is
eventually entered into CANCERPROJ, one of the files which comprise
the CANCERLINE Data Base. Epidemiological studies concerning chemicals are notified to the Information Bulletin of the Survey of
Chemicals Being Tested for Carcinogenicity, published by IARC, so
that workers in the field of experimental carcinogenesis can be aware
of human exposures.

While there is increasing interest in cancer epidemiology and a belief that research effort in this area needs to be greatly expanded,
no attempt has to our knowledge been made to quantify, however
crudely, what is being done in the various parts of the world. This
paper thus analyses the nature and geographical distribution of
studies reported to the CH in 1977 (Muir & Wagner, 1977), and further
comments on some of the existing impediments to epidemiological
cancer research which are considered to be currently operating.

METHODS AND MATERIAL

Each of the studies appearing in the 1977 Directory of On-going
Research in Cancer Epidemiology were assigned to one or, very rarely,
two broad categories, these being :

        a) Case-control studies (CAC). This category included
studies using the case-control method ; but those case-control
studies examining, say, a viral hypothesis of aetiology were allocated to VIRUS (See k) below. This method of allocation results in
an underestimation of the frequency of the use of the case-control
method.

        b) Case characteristics (CCH). This category comprised
reports of the characteristics of patients with specific cancers
but for whom there was no control group. These studies were included
in the directory as the information derived may be useful for hypothesis formulation.

       c) Correlation (CORR). This category was used for studies
comparing population characteristics with cancer frequency at the
group level. For example, pesticide levels and malignant lymphoma
incidence in several countries or within a country.

       d) Genetic or familial (GEN). This category included stu-
dies of cancer family trees, HLA distribution in cancer patients and
the like.

       e) High-risk groups (HIR). This category excluded indus-
trial high-risk groups (INDU, see f) below and those with radiation
exposure (RADIAT, see h) below. A prospective study of takers of a
particular drug or a cohort of alcoholics, for example, would be
included in this category.

       f) Industrial (INDU). This category concerned industrial
exposures other than radiation (RADIAT) and largely dealt with exposure to specific chemicals or group of chemicals.

       g) Morphological (MORPH). This category included investi-
gations relating morphology (histology) to aetiology. For example,
the relation between the histological types of lung cancer and
smoking.

       h) Radiation exposure (RADIAT). This category was confined
to examination of the consequences of exposure to ionizing radiation.

       i) Screening (SCREEN). This category pertained to those
screening studies which contained an element of evaluation.

       j) Statistics (STAT). This category was used for studies
of a statistical nature, for example, mortality, incidence, time
trends and relative frequency.

       k) Virological (VIRUS). This category was reserved for
epidemiological studies, no matter how conducted, testing the virus
hypothesis of cancer aetiology.

Similarly, the primary sites of cancer under study were assigned
either to the organ in question or to a group of organs. When the
same study dealt with more than one anatomical site which involved
several systems of the body, these were considered separately. For
cohort studies, for example, an increased risk of cancer at any site
is of interest and hence the category "all sites" is frequently
used.

RESULTS

A total of 1087 cancer sites relating to 908 projects in cancer epidemiology were categorized in the manner described above. In
Table 1, the various broad study categories are examined by country
or region. Studies were reported from 70 countries : over half were
from four countries, the USA : 32.4%, the United Kingdom : 13.8%,
Canada : 5.3%, Japan : 4.1%.

Statistical studies, largely descriptive, accounted for 18.8%, the
health effects of industrial exposures 16.3%, case-control studies
14.9% and correlation studies 12.8%. There are considerable differ-

ences in the frequency of study type by region.   Case-control studies were relatively few in Africa, Australia and East Europe, the
evaluation of industrial risk was frequent in Canada and in the
United Kingdom as were statistical studies in Africa and South
America.

The type of investigation undertaken has also been cross-tabulated
with the various cancer sites (Table 2).   The information in both
tables is rather simplistic in that for the vast majority only one
study type was allocated to each investigation.   For many investigations, notably those of a statistical nature and cohort studies involving high risk or industrial groups, cancer arising in any organ
is of interest and "All Sites" comprises the largest category in the
table.   Case-control studies were frequently used to study breast,
urinary tract, large intestine, malignant lymphoma and leukaemia.
For many industrial studies the lung was the suspect target organ.
The viral hypothesis was investigated most frequently for nasopharynx, cervix uteri and malignant lymphoma.   Correlation studies were
frequent in relation to lung, breast and stomach.   Despite their
present numerical importance and the fact that they seem to be increasing in many parts of the world, even in populations where these
neoplasms have hitherto been considered to be rare, there is practically no work on pancreas, prostate or malignant melanoma.

DISCUSSION

It must be repeated that the analyses contained in Tables 1 and 2
are over-simplifications of a complex situation.   It is probable
that the CH does not receive information from a considerable proportion of investigators, and further the degree of such under-report-
ing may vary from country to country, or even within a country. Con-
versely, the CH policy has been to define epidemiology fairly broadly and it could thus be argued that the Annual Directory published
by the CH over-estimates the amount of epidemiological work under-
way.   Nonetheless, to our knowledge, this paper constitutes a first
attempt to assess the current level and scope of epidemiological
activity in cancer.

The amount of information provided by contributors to the CH varied
greatly.   Some give the range of data normally appearing in a summary
of a research grant application - others are very cryptic :   Smith
(1978) has suggested that original ideas are unlikely to find their
first expression in such a CH.   Smith further suggested that investigators be asked in future to give the number of patients to be studied as this would in some instances give a measure, if but crude,
of the potential usefulness of the study.   The editors concur but
are well aware of the danger of antagonizing respondents by asking
for too much information.   Nonetheless, many scientists have willing-
ly provided the editors with further details about their work when
needed.   Studies of industrial hazards pose particular problems as
some investigators consider that to mention a chemical or industry
before the study is complete may impair the successful and impartial
assessment of the risk.   In assessing the nature of the epidemiological work being conducted, the assignment of but one study type to an
investigation is bound to result in some distortion, as does grouping of cancer sites.

Whatever the failings of the CH, the analysis of Tables 1 and 2 indicates that epidemiological effort is globally uneven and that
many numerically important cancers are receiving scant attention.
Some of the barriers to epidemiological research which we believe
to exist are considered below.

Barriers To Epidemiological Research

While it is possible that a knowledge of the mechanisms of carcinogenesis may eventually lead to methods to prevent cancer, this is
not for the immediate future and rational cancer control is likely
to depend for at least the next decade on determining the aetiology
of the disease. The discovery of causal factors, whether these be
exposure to some chemical or aspects of diet or "lifestyle",
implies the availability of both mechanisms to facilitate detection
and of trained personnel to carry out the work. All over the world
both areas are in need of considerable improvement.

Record linkage. While the causes of cancer can be elucidated by
many approaches, the cohort study, retrospective or prospective,
is among the more important.

The key to the economical identification of risk lies in the ability
to assemble cohorts of exposed persons and then follow them up to
death, or preferably, their appearance in the files of a cancer
registry. This implies the ability to unequivocally link an individual on two sets of records and to have access, not necessarily
nominal, to cancer registry files or to the medical cause of death
given on the death certificate. Absolute secrecy of the death certificate such as exists in several European countries, and an inability to match data sets ensure that risk remains undetected.

Manpower and training. There is probably no part of the world in
which it is not possible to conduct valid epidemiological studies.
These may range from assessment of the relative frequency of cancer
in clinical or pathology records through case-control studies to
complex cohort investigations. The simpler studies need not be
undertaken by an epidemiologist but those doing them should have
access to the advice of an epidemiologist trained in chronic disease
epidemiology.

Cancer epidemiology is currently undertaken by a wide variety of
bodies including specialized units created by research councils,
and university and government departments, as well as by individuals.
The recruitment and training of epidemiologists is often haphazard
and there is rarely a career structure with a clearly defined number
of established positions as exists for, say, pathology.

The concept of epidemiology varies widely in different parts of the
world. In the USSR, it is essentially "the science of the objective
laws underlying the origin, spread and decline of infectious disease
in human population groups, and of the prophylaxis and eradication
of these diseases". More recently, this definition has been broaden-
ed. Clearly, the use of epidemiological methods of research and
study of non-infectious diseases, while quite justified, does not
imply an expansion of the subject matter of epidemiology as a science
and, therefore, the use of the term for other purposes is purely

optional and cannot be considered as strictly "scientific". In the
United Kingdom, on the other hand, it is common to regard epidemiology as "a set of techniques" that can be applied to a large range
of problems encountered in the different aspects of medical practice.
Such differences in interpretation give rise to wide differences in
teaching between those medical schools that restrict their courses
to communicable diseases and those that devote at least as much time
to the epidemiology of non-communicable diseases, disabilities and
accidents. In between are faculties that give a more or less full
course on the classical epidemiology of infectious diseases and
graft on to this a brief study of the epidemiology of non-communicable disease. Very broadly, these three divisions are characteristic of teaching in eastern Europe, north-west Europe and central and
southern Europe respectively (Cottrel, Kesic and Senault, 1969).

In their publication "The Teaching of Public Health in Europe",
Cottrel, Kesic and Senault reviewed the situation in each country,
and suggested that chronic disease epidemiology should be more
widely taught in European medical schools. A similar survey should
be repeated not only in Europe but in other parts of the world to
determine the current situation. Although excellent texts exist
(Lowe and Kostrewski, 1973), unfortunately the undergraduate con-
siders as serious only those subjects which are linked to an academic department and an examination. Such an academic department
need not necessarily be a chair of epidemiology per se but the discipline should be strongly represented in a University Department of
Public Health and Community Medicine. If epidemiology is to advance,
this academic infrastructure must be created first.

CONCLUSION

Analysis of the studies notified to the Clearing House of On-going
Research in Cancer Epidemiology shows that although much useful epidemiological work in cancer could be undertaken in most of the world,
effort seems currently to be concentrated in U.S., U.K., Canada and
Japan. Further, little work is being done on numerically important
cancer, such as malignant melanoma, prostate and pancreas. Finance
apart, the major barriers to epidemiological research are considered
to be lack of trained manpower, a lack possibly influenced by differing national concepts of the nature and the potential of epidemiology,
and the inability to easily link an exposure and its subsequent health
effects in the individual. The investment in epidemiological effort
in the world today is trivial in relation to study opportunities and
needs.

REFERENCES

Cottrel, J.D., B. Kesic, and R. Senault (1969). The Teaching of Public Health in Europe. World Health Organization : Monograph Series No. 58, 246 p.

Lowe, C.R., and J. Kostrewski (1973). A Guide to Teaching Methods. International Epidemiological Association. Churchill/Livingston, London and Edinburgh.

Muir, C.S., and G. Wagner, (Ed.) (1976). Directory of On-going Research in Cancer Epidemiology, International Agency for Research on Cancer, Lyon, and Deutsches Krebsforschungszentrum, Heidelberg.

Muir, C.S., and G. Wagner (Ed.) (1977). Directory of On-going Research in Cancer Epidemiology, Lyon, International Agency for Research on Cancer (IARC Scientific Publications No. 17).

Muir, C.S., and G. Wagner (Ed.) (1978). Directory of On-going Research in Cancer Epidemiology, International Agency for Research on Cancer (IARC Scientific Publications No. 26).

Smith, P.G. (1978). Book Review. Br. J. Cancer, 38, 206.

Index

The page numbers refer to the first page of the article in which the index term appears.